"Terry Lemerond is the most healthy, energetic, positive and spiritually sound person I know. Read this book and learn how he does it." Siri Khalsa, Editor of *Nutrition News*

"Terry is a role model and inspiration to all. His book should be mandatory reading for everyone, but especially doctors. If all doctors would espouse the principles in Terry's book to all their patients, there would be a tremendous decrease in sickness and disease and a huge increase in the quality of everyone's life."

Jan McBarron, M.D.

"Terry Lemerond has written a book which belongs in the hands of every person who wants to know how to enjoy life to the fullest."

Robert C. Martin, D.C., Clinical Nutritionist, National Syndicated Host of *Health Talk*

"As you go through life, many decisions you make will affect your health. In **Seven Keys to Vibrant Health,** *Terry Lemerond teaches you how to live your life in a manner that will maximize your potential for wellness. This is a book that can change your life for the better—not only by keeping you healthy, but also by showing you how you can live a life of personal fulfillment."* Melvyn R. Werbach, M.D.

"Finally, a most practical book for all people who want to be healthy, avoid the killer diseases and slow the aging process."

Arnold Fox, M.D.

"Terry Lemerond has been a major inspiration in my life as well as the lives of many others. He is a man of high principles who actually adheres to them. In other words, Terry walks his talk. As a result, he is a living testimony to the powerful impact that the keys outlined in this book can have on a person's life."

Michael T. Murray, N.D.

"Seven Keys to Vibrant Health *is a landmark, a guidepost! It provides the reader with a simple method to live a healthier, happier, longer, more pain-free life. Each chapter is a jewel. I found myself going back to the book, over and over again.*"   Anthony J. Cichoke, M.A., D.C., D.A.C.B.N.

"*...must-reading for every household...*"

Earl Mindell, Ph.D., author of *The Vitamin Bible*

"*Certainly will help rejuvenate anyone!*"

Devra Hill, Ph.D., author of *Rejuvenate*

"*...a great book on negotiating optimum health...*"

Riki Robbins Jones, Ph.D., author of *Negotiating Love*

"*Gives us deep insight into ourselves—enriching us all.*"

Willie Southall, author of *Hyssop: Superior Healing Power*

"*...unlocks the secrets of optimum health...*"

Dick Quinn, author of *Left for Dead*

"*Terry Lemerond is a gentleman, a scholar, and an altruist. His book is an invaluable collection of scientifically proven tips on extending the quality and quantity of life while preventing and even reversing disease. America would spring into a new era of wellness and prosperity if these principles were adopted.*"

Patrick Quillin, Ph.D., R.D., CNS, author of 8 books and
Vice President of Nutrition for Cancer Treatment Centers of America

Seven Keys to Vibrant Health

by

Terry Lemerond

President of Enzymatic Therapy

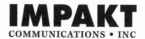
IMPAKT
COMMUNICATIONS • INC

P.O. Box 12496
Green Bay, WI 54307-2496
(414) 499-2995

Cover design and photos by: *Dawn Sandve*
Copyediting by: *Lara Pizzorno, Betty Leneau, John Robinson*
Production and interior design by: *Kelly Fisher*

Library of Congress Catalog Card Number: 95-78606
ISBN 0-9647489-0-8

PRINTED IN THE UNITED STATES OF AMERICA

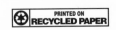

DEDICATION

This book is dedicated to my family:
Brad and Stephanie Lemerond, Teppie and Matt Schueller, and especially
my mother, who gave me the chance to start my journey

TABLE OF CONTENTS

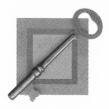

xi   *Foreword by Michael T. Murray, N.D.*
xiii   *Preface*
xiv   *Introduction*

CHAPTER 1. KEY #1—SPIRITUALITY

2   STEP 1. *Realize the power of prayer*
4   STEP 2. *Make prayer part of your daily routine*
4   STEP 3. *Read the Bible*
6   STEP 4. *Use the power of love*
7   STEP 5. *Become a servant of others*
8   STEP 6. *Tithe*
9   STEP 7. *Attend church regularly*

CHAPTER 2. KEY #2—POSITIVE ATTITUDE

12   STEP 1. *Become an optimist*
24   STEP 2. *Practice positive self-talk*
24   STEP 3. *Ask better questions*
26   STEP 4. *Employ positive affirmations*
27   STEP 5. *Set positive goals*
28   STEP 6. *Use positive visualization*
31   STEP 7. *Read or listen to positive messages*

CHAPTER 3. KEY #3—POSITIVE RELATIONSHIPS

38   STEP 1. *Learn to help others*
40   STEP 2. *Develop positive qualities*
41   STEP 3. *Learn to listen*
43   STEP 4. *Find the good*
44   STEP 5. *Demonstrate love and appreciation*
44   STEP 6. *Develop intimacy*
46   STEP 7. *Recognize challenges in relationships*

CHAPTER 4. KEY #4—A HEALTHY LIFESTYLE

50   STEP 1. *Do not smoke*

52   STEP 2. *Do not drink or drink only in moderation*

53   STEP 3. *Get adequate rest*

54   STEP 4. *Learn to deal with stress effectively*

56   STEP 5. *Learn to manage time effectively*

58   STEP 6. *Connect with nature*

58   STEP 7. *Laugh long and often*

CHAPTER 5. KEY #5—REGULAR EXERCISE

67   STEP 1. *Realize the importance of physical exercise*

67   STEP 2. *Consult your physician*

68   STEP 3. *Select an activity you can enjoy*

68   STEP 4. *Monitor your exercise intensity*

69   STEP 5. *Do it often*

69   STEP 6. *Make it fun*

69   STEP 7. *Stay motivated*

CHAPTER 6. KEY #6—A HEALTH-PROMOTING DIET

76   STEP 1. *Reduce your fat intake*

76   STEP 2. *Eat five or more servings of vegetables and fruits daily*

76   STEP 3. *Limit your refined sugar intake*

77   STEP 4. *Increase your fiber and complex carbohydrate intake*

78   STEP 5. *Maintain protein intake at moderate levels*

78   STEP 6. *Limit your salt intake*

79   STEP 7. *Take time for menu planning*

CHAPTER 7. KEY #7—SUPPLEMENTATION

85   STEP 1. *Take a high-potency multiple vitamin and mineral formula*

87   STEP 2. *Take additional antioxidants*

90   STEP 3. *Use formulas designed to support specific body functions*

92   STEP 4. *Use glandular support*

95   STEP 5. *Use purified, standardized botanical extracts*

102 STEP 6. *Use homeopathic medicines*

104 STEP 7. *Use natural medicines*

ACKNOWLEDGEMENTS

I would like to express my love and gratitude to the many people who offered their guidance, encouragement, valuable support, and friendship over the years that I developed and refined my personal health beliefs.

To **Michael Murray, N.D.**, because of his unique talent in making sense out of, and putting into written form, our numerous conversations and dozens of tapings, and who knows my philosophies better than anyone else.

To **Lara Pizzorno**, for her wonderful skill in editing the book to its final form.

To **Dawn Sandve**, for her very creative and beautiful cover that gives meaning to the "Seven Keys."

To **John Robinson**, for his input on some of the more critical chapters.

To **Frances FitzGerald**, for assisting me with her creative writing skills, allowing me to say the things I needed to say in this book.

To my family at **Enzymatic Therapy, PhytoPharmica, Bay Natural Nutritionals,** and *Prescription For Health*. These wonderful people have supported my dreams and goals and have helped make them possible. Without these dedicated people, this book would not have been possible.

And of course, thanks to my family—**Brad, Stephanie, Teppie, and Matt**—who are always there for me and allow me to be just who I am.

And last of all, but most important, I thank **God** for His guidance and blessings, for He has always been the center of my life, both personally and in business. This book and my journey could not have been possible without the love and care I feel from God. I cannot claim to have the skills or the talents to take credit for the success that has blessed my life. Truly, God has touched me in a way that I can only praise and thank Him for every day of my life.

FOREWORD

Terry Lemerond has been a major inspiration in my life as well as the lives of many others. He is a man of high principles who actually adheres to them. In other words—Terry walks his talk. As a result, he is a living testimony to the powerful impact that adhering to the "keys" outlined in his book can have on a person's life.

When I first met Terry in late September of 1985, I had just graduated from Bastyr University in Seattle, Washington, with a degree in naturopathic medicine. Terry had just started Enzymatic Therapy which, at the time, was a very small company in the natural health industry. Terry was looking for some technical support for his company. Dr. Joseph Pizzorno and I had just completed the first edition of *A Textbook of Natural Medicine*. Based on this work, Terry felt I had the type of technical expertise that could help his company.

Have you ever met someone and felt as if you had known him all your life? A cliché, I know, but when I met Terry I immediately experienced a deep feeling of recognition. The more we talked and learned about each other, the more I understood our immediate bond. We shared many of the same values, principles, beliefs, and philosophies. We had a lot in common.

As we each shared our vision of what we wanted to see in the natural health movement, it became obvious to us both that we were destined to help one another improve the lives of others. One of the things I wanted to see was high-quality herbal products standardized for their potency. During my research on *A Textbook of Natural Medicine*, I kept coming across studies on some phenomenal herbal products that were not yet available in the United States. It was frustrating to me that Americans did not have access to high-quality herbal products like the standardized extracts of Ginkgo biloba, saw palmetto, and milk thistle available in Europe. I knew the benefits these herbal extracts possessed and had shared this information with many companies in the natural food industry, but these other companies could not embrace my vision. Instead, they focused on all the tremendous obstacles. Terry was different; he had the same vision I did.

It has been extremely gratifying for us both to see much of our vision for natural products in the United States become reality. It warms our hearts to know that people are receiving benefits from the many products—like ginkgo, glucosamine sulfate, saw palmetto, DGL, and enteric-coated peppermint oil—that Enzymatic Therapy has introduced to America.

Have you ever seen *The Blues Brothers*—a movie with John Belushi and Dan Akroyd? Terry and I joke about being on a similar mission from God. We may kid one another about our mission, but we both genuinely feel it is our duty to help people achieve greater health and happiness in their lives. I know this sense of mission is what drives Terry. It drives him to produce the highest quality natural products in the world, and it is what has driven him to write this book.

I know firsthand the type of man Terry Lemerond is. Over the years, I have witnessed his unwavering integrity, kindness, generosity, honesty, and loyalty. He is a man who lives his religion. It is my hope that reading his book will give you a glimpse of the spirit that informs his life. I am truly honored to call him my friend.

I also hope that you will put the *Seven Keys to Vibrant Health* to work in your life. This book will not only help you achieve greater health, but also greater happiness and passion. Life is a wonderful gift; Terry's book will help you to make the most of it!

Michael T. Murray, N.D.

PREFACE

Dear Reader:

The reason I decided to write this book is to share an insight that took me years to discover for myself: *We can choose the kind of lives we want to live.* When we start making conscious choices about our spirituality, attitude, relationships, lifestyle habits, exercise, diet and supplementation—we come closer to achieving vibrant health and enduring happiness.

Why should you listen to me? After all, I'm not a doctor or a psychologist or even a professional writer. I was not born into wealth or privilege; I was not blessed with extraordinary genius. What I do have is a lifelong passion for natural health and self-empowerment. I don't believe our health and our lives are determined for us—I believe *we* determine what they will be.

It isn't easy. Change means giving up familiar ways of thinking and eating and interacting with others. And you've got a lot to lose: a negative attitude, loneliness, hopelessness, bad habits, fatigue, and sluggish health. Of course, if you feel you'd be better off without these things, then maybe you're ready for change. I can promise you that once you make these changes, you'll never look back.

When you work on each important area of your life, you'll find they work together to create a greater whole. For example, when you exercise, you improve your mood, which fosters a more positive attitude. When you develop meaningful relationships, you are more motivated to take care of your body through a healthful diet. They are all interrelated; and as one area unfolds, it touches and enriches every other area of your life.

My company has enjoyed great success with nutritional and botanical supplements and natural medicines. But I didn't get into this business to turn a profit. I chose this enterprise because I want people like you to enjoy extraordinary health, and perhaps more importantly, I want you to realize you can do it for yourself.

By opening this book, you have just taken an important step. May God bless you with health, prosperity, and success.

Terrence J. Lemerond
January, 1995

INTRODUCTION

Seven Keys to Vibrant Health provides a blueprint for health that I have seen work miracles in my life and the lives of others. I did not "discover" these keys; people who are truly healthy simply possess these traits. My belief is that if you or I can also possess these keys, we, too, can achieve more health in our lives.

Your life can be better if you follow the guidelines described in this book. No matter where you are in life—old or young, rich or poor, no matter what your personal history or education level—you can always get better from the moment you decide to improve. Making the decision to get better is the number one step to a life filled with more health, happiness, passion, and joy.

As is the case in achieving anything we desire in life, we first have to decide what it is that we truly want. Do you really want to have greater health in life? How would you feel if you possessed vibrant, radiant health and energy? Once we really become focused on what it is we want, the next steps involve unlocking the keys to achieve our goal.

The farmer can decide to plant the seed, but before he plants, he must have some tools. He has to cultivate the land, he has to till the soil, he has to fertilize the soil. He must do many things to prepare the earth before he plants the seed. Planting an idea or goal in a human being is a similar process. We can't just plant the seed. We must use the right tools to cultivate it, to nurture the seed so it will grow. Those tools come in the form of patience, faith, and tenacity, of perseverance when we fear the seed won't germinate. The farmer, when he plants the seed, doesn't sit and fret and worry that the seed isn't going to come up. He knows from past experience that, without some unforeseen natural catastrophe, a properly nurtured seed will germinate.

I've learned over the years that the same scenario applies to the human experience. The seed of a goal or dream will germinate, but we need to have the faith, the patience, the tenacity, and the perseverance to believe it will grow and just work in good faith.

So many times, I have seen people give up on their goals or dreams, especially regarding health, before they have really given them a chance. They lose faith. I like to tell people the story of the bamboo tree because it is such a beautiful example of the power of diligence.

A village received a seed of the bamboo tree as a gift from a neighboring village. They were told to plant it, water it, and care for it, so it would grow to a great size and provide shade from the hot sun for the village. The villagers planted the seed and cared for it for one full year, but nothing happened. Many of the villagers wanted to give up. "Why should we work so hard to care for this seed when it is obvious that it is dead and will never grow?" one of them asked the chief of the village. The chief, a man of great faith, trusted the seed would eventually grow to a great bamboo tree. He was able to paint the picture in the minds of all the villagers of how magnificent it would be when the bamboo tree reached maturity. Because of the power of his faith and vision, the villagers continued to work hard, despite the fact that nothing happened for over four years. Finally, during the fifth year, a sprout started to come through the soil. A miracle was proclaimed when, just ninety days after the first sprout, the chief's vision—a ninety-foot bamboo tree—became a reality.

Why did it take five years before any evidence appeared that the seed had germinated? While nothing was apparent above the ground, in the soil a very extensive root system was developing to provide the kind of support that would allow the bamboo shoots to grow at an amazing rate—a foot a day. In order to support such growth, the seed, in all its wisdom, was growing downward rather than upward to form the huge foundation of root systems necessary.

To achieve good health, you, too, must develop a strong foundation. This takes time. Many people with whom I have come into contact believe that, after abusing themselves for 20-30 years, they can simply take a bottle of something for a month, put together some sort of health or nutritional program, go on a weight loss program, or exercise for a couple of weeks, and reverse all the years of abuse. When they don't see an obvious improvement after a month or so, they become discouraged and quit. What they don't realize is that they're building a strong foundation. If they persevere, once they reach a certain point, it's just like the bamboo tree: growth is exponential.

The human body is constantly regenerating. Because the cells in our bodies are continually changing, we can create a whole new self over time. For example, every three to four days, we gain a whole new lining in the gastrointestinal tract as new cells are formed to replace damaged old cells. In just thirty days, we renew our entire skin, and every six weeks, we make an entirely new liver. We live within the most amazing piece of machinery. (I don't like to use the word machinery, but use it for lack of a better word.) We can be very abusive to our body, yet it is very forgiving. If you give your body enough time, you can actually recreate your entire system.

So often I see people start a new health or weight loss program but then give up far too early. Don't give up. I have seen the seven keys to vibrant health work wonders in my own life. Follow these keys, and you will achieve a healthier life. Believe it, because it is true.

When I was growing up, I was fortunate (or unfortunate) to have access to many things that weren't good for me. Junk foods, candies and soft drinks became the major staples of my diet. As a young man of 20, I weighed over 200 pounds. At a height of 5'6", I was nearly as wide around as I was tall. In addition to being fat, I also had very severe hypoglycemia which resulted in a lot of mental, emotional, and behavioral problems due to the severe mood swings caused by my erratically plummeting blood sugar levels.

Because of my unruly behavior and attitude, I was not a very well-liked person. I knew my life was in trouble, so I gave up three years of college to join the Marine Corps. I wanted to see if they could "make a man out of me."

Joining the Marine Corps definitely changed my life for the better. Perhaps the best thing that happened to me was meeting Captain Ed Vito, who helped me learn the value of good health and proper nutrition.

I met Captain Vito when I joined the weight-lifting team after boot camp. I had lost a lot of weight during boot camp—a side effect of twelve weeks of continuous calisthenics, obstacle courses, marching and running. I was definitely in better shape, but didn't have good muscle tone, so I joined the weight-lifting team.

Captain Vito was knowledgeable not only about weight-lifting but also about nutrition. I was very fortunate to be taken under his wing and introduced to the tremendous value of proper nutrition.

When he took me home on weekends, I saw the healthful diet he and his family ate. Their diet focused on fresh fruits and vegetables, whole grains, sprouts, and a lot of other foods I had never eaten in any quantity.

Captain Vito also took me to a health food store for the very first time—a small store in Oceanside, California, during 1959. At that time, health food stores were much smaller than they are today. There were few products on the shelves, but a lot more than I had ever seen.

With Captain Vito's introduction, I became completely fascinated with health. I noticed that as I became healthier, I became much happier. My mood swings disappeared, and I felt better about life than I ever had. As my muscle tone improved, I looked healthier than I ever had. When I returned to Green Bay in 1962 after my stint in the Marines, people didn't recognize the man I had become.

I was extremely excited about what health foods, good nutrition and vitamins could do. When I left, Green Bay had no health food stores, so I was delighted when I looked in the Yellow Pages to discover a store called Bay Natural Foods had opened up. Immediately, I went down and introduced myself to the owner, Claire Delsmann. A delightful lady who had never married, Claire built the store by treating her customers like family.

Eventually, the store grew until it became too much for Claire to handle alone. I found myself helping her out for free before I went to work and on weekends, because I loved the store and was so glad it was available in Green Bay. I was working nights at a machine shop but would drop by the store in the morning just to say hello. I worked for Claire for about seven years, part-time, free. I ran the store for her when she was on vacation. When she took a day off, I'd come in at 9:00 a.m. and work until a couple of minutes to 3:00 p.m., then run across town to the machine shop.

Finally, in 1969, Claire just couldn't run the store anymore. She had to sell but wanted somebody who shared her philosophy and would continue to run it like an extended family. This store was Claire's "baby." She wanted to make sure it was loved and nurtured.

Claire knew how much I loved the store. I was there all the time. When you love someone you want to be there, you want to touch them, you want to hold them, you want to know everything that you can about them. Strange as it may sound, this was the kind of love I had for Bay Natural Foods. So, I was there all the time. I would stop in before work, after work, in between, any time I had a chance, I would go to help Claire or to read.

Claire wanted someone with that kind of dedication to take over the store, but I didn't have the money, so selling to me just didn't make sense. Finally, she found a person who had the money and wanted to buy the store, but she wasn't comfortable selling to a stranger. So, on a Saturday afternoon in February 1969, the course of my life changed forever.

Claire usually closed the store at noon on Saturdays. On this particular Saturday, however, I was staying late to paint the walls and spruce the store up a bit. Claire began telling me her dreams and what she wanted to see happen to the store. When I replied, "That's great. I support you 100%. I want that to happen for you, and I hope it does," she said, "Well, it can, if someone buys the store who has the same philosophy I have." When I said, "I agree with you completely," she asked, "Terry, why don't you buy the store?"

I explained to Claire that although owning Bay Natural Foods would be a dream come true, I didn't have any money. I couldn't see how it would be possible. Claire's desire for me to buy the store was so great, she decided to help me. With Claire's help, as well as some help from my mother and the bank, I was able to raise enough cash to buy the store.

From 1969 to 1981, I worked in Bay Natural Foods educating people about the value of good nutrition and proper nutritional supplementation. Through years of study and experience, I had learned that certain vitamins, minerals, herbs, and glandular concentrates would produce far better results when combined than when they were taken individually. Rather than sending people home with a dozen different bottles of supplements, I wanted to use formulas that combined the essential nutrients and support to meet my clients' specific nutritional needs. I had a dream: a company that would develop and sell state-of-the art nutritional and botanical products designed to support specific body functions. In 1981, this company—Enzymatic Therapy—was born.

Enzymatic Therapy began with ten products. I selected only the highest quality raw materials regardless of their cost because I knew the measure of my success would be the results my clients experienced. As word spread of my formulas and their effectiveness, Enzymatic Therapy began offering these products to health food stores across the country.

Like the bamboo tree, in the last ten years, Enzymatic Therapy has become one of the fastest growing companies in the natural foods industry. Currently, Enzymatic Therapy offers over 180 innovative products, advances in nutritional supplementation which are the concrete embodiment of our desire for you to get results.

As a result of our commitment to providing the absolute best products, Enzymatic Therapy has established itself as the leader in the industry. I am so proud of our long list of industry firsts. Enzymatic Therapy was the first company in the United States to introduce standardized herbal extracts, phytosomes, and predigested glandular concentrates. Here is just a partial list of products we have introduced to Americans:

- Ginkgo biloba extract
- Glucosamine sulfate
- Silymarin
- Enteric-coated peppermint oil
- Bilberry extract
- DGL (deglycyrrhizinated licorice)
- Saw palmetto berry extract

The growth and success of Enzymatic Therapy is based on the company's adherence to the same keys which are detailed in this book.

I hope you enjoy *Seven Keys to Vibrant Health*. I pray that it will answer some of your questions about health and will help inspire you to lead a life filled with vibrant health and happiness.

Terry Lemerond
President of Enzymatic Therapy

CHAPTER ONE

KEY #1—SPIRITUALITY

STEP 1.
Realize the power of prayer

STEP 2.
Make prayer part of your daily routine

STEP 3.
Read the Bible

STEP 4.
Use the power of love

STEP 5.
Become a servant of others

STEP 6.
Tithe

STEP 7.
Attend church regularly

KEY #1—SPIRITUALITY

Spirituality means different things to different people. For me, it means doing my best to emulate the teachings of Jesus. I am a Christian. I know non-Christians may have a different faith that is just as strong and just as valid. Some people may not conceptualize a personal God, yet hold a sense of godliness and sacredness in their everyday lives.

Please understand that when I talk about my spiritual beliefs, I am in no way trying to claim religious superiority or exclusivity. I believe that God—however or whatever you imagine God to be—works in our lives for good. And I believe God can have a profound effect on our health.

I've been in the natural health business for the past 25 years: first as a health food store retailer, then as president and founder of Enzymatic Therapy, a manufacturer of nutritional and botanical supplements. I've spoken with thousands of people about their experiences with conventional and non-conventional therapies, with mainstream physicians and alternative practitioners, with prescription medicines and natural supplements.

I've reached the conclusion that the most powerful medicine of all may have nothing to do with drugs, surgery, or other medical "magic bullets." I have seen for myself that the human spirit is phenomenally therapeutic and can create miracles when science falls short.

STEP 1. *Realize the power of prayer*

Prayer is especially good medicine. Consider the study by cardiologist Randolph Byrd, published in the *Southern Medical Journal* in 1986. Over a period of ten months, Dr. Byrd investigated almost 400 patients in the coronary care unit at San Francisco's General Hospital.

In this randomized, double-blind study, one group of patients was prayed for by home prayer groups, while the other group was not. The people who prayed were given a brief description of each patient's ailment. Each patient in the prayed-for group had between five and seven people praying for him or her. Neither the patients, nor the doctors, nor the nurses knew who was in which group.

After ten months, Byrd found the following differences between the two groups:

- The prayed-for patients were five times less likely to need antibiotic medication.
- The prayed-for patients were three times less likely to have their lungs fill with fluid (pulmonary edema).
- None of the prayed-for patients needed to be on mechanical ventilators. In contrast, 12 of the unprayed-for patients needed help breathing.
- Fewer of the prayed-for group died.

Larry Dossey, M.D., co-chairman of the National Institutes of Health's Office of Alternative Medicine and author of *Healing Words*, said, "The evidence is simply overwhelming that prayer functions at a distance to change physical processes in a variety of organisms, from bacteria to humans" (as quoted in "Why Prayer is Great Medicine" by Mary Ellen Hettinger, published in *Your Health*).

If praying is good for others, can we do it for ourselves? Absolutely. Herbert Benson, M.D., founding president of the Mind/Body Medical Institute, in Boston, Massachusetts, studied the physiological changes that prayer could set into motion. He found that patients who prayed and/or meditated could elicit a relaxation response. This response includes a decrease in heart rate, breathing rate, muscle tension, and sometimes even blood pressure.

What are the medical implications? This relaxation response could have a beneficial impact on cases of hypertension, muscle tension pain, headaches, infertility, insomnia, psychological distress, cardiac arrhythmias, premenstrual syndrome, and symptoms of cancer and AIDS.

You may be thinking God has less to do with this effect than we do. You may believe the healing comes from within ourselves, not from "up above." But I feel that within us is exactly where God resides, and that when we pray and meditate, we unleash God's power.

Scientists are just beginning to look into the healing potential of prayer. Fortunately, we don't have to wait for controlled studies, published reports, or FDA approval to use prayer in our everyday lives. Prayer is absolutely safe and is available to each of us, whenever we wish to make use of it.

Prayer costs nothing, hurts nothing, and works on many levels. It fits perfectly into any treatment plan. No matter what your particular faith, prayer can lead you to greater health—of body, mind, and soul.

STEP 2. *Make prayer part of your daily routine*

Prayer, to me, means communion with God. While formal verbal prayers are nice, I prefer to pray in silence. Rather than recite a hundred Hail Marys, I place myself in a silent state, get in touch with my inner being, and speak to God.

I ask God to help me or whomever I am praying for. The Bible says, "You have not because you ask not...Ask and you will receive."

Between the asking and the receiving is a period of waiting— time in which, I believe, God tests our faith and trust. God has a season for all things, and God can be trusted to act in the right time. Once we ask, then we have to put away all cares and all worries and just know that it has been done.

It is also important to ask with gratitude. You never ask anyone for something without saying thank you. So when you pray, do so with gratitude to God for answering your prayer.

Set aside at least 20 to 30 minutes a day for prayer. That 20 to 30 minutes a day not only will give you the opportunity to communicate with your Creator and with yourself, but also you will find that in those minutes you'll discover new ideas, new things you never thought about, and answers to problems. They'll start coming to you because you have allowed yourself this quiet time. When we quiet ourselves, we open up the communication lines to our inner self and God. We aren't asking questions anymore, we aren't trying to think of things, we are just letting ourselves become open for information. A conversation should be two-way; we aren't just asking from God, we are also receiving. Prayer is a time when you are leaving your mind wide open.

STEP 3. *Read the Bible*

Being a Christian, I try to read something from the Bible daily. I know this has had a powerful influence in my life. God is my Creator. He put me on this earth, and I don't think God would put me here without giving me some instructions. When we buy an appliance, we get a manual that teaches us how to use the appliance. When God put us on this earth, I believe He gave us a manual as well—the Bible. It holds all the instructions of good living: how to sow and reap, how to tithe, how to be respectful of one another, how to be a good steward, and how to be a servant, because the servant is the one who is exalted. The Bible provides the guidelines for being a good Christian. To me, being a Christian doesn't just mean what ideas I believe in. It describes the way I try to treat my family, my friends, and my employees. It's the way I try to do business. It's the way I try to live my life. I don't always succeed, but I keep striving toward these Christian standards.

The Bible gives us so many examples which clearly teach us how to live with spirituality. I have a rather broad definition of spirituality. To me it means expressing everything good that we have in our being—faith, love, hope, honor, integrity, etc. I believe that spirituality is God working through me. Spirituality is all that God brings within me, and the Bible is my guide for accessing God within me.

One of the passages in the Bible that has helped me immensely is from Proverbs 3:5-6, "Trust in the Lord with all your heart and lean not on your own understanding; in all your ways acknowledge Him, and He will make your path straight."

Sometimes things happen in our lives, and we don't understand why they happen. The Bible says that "All things happen for good to those who love the Lord." I really believe this. And, when it says "all things," it means not just some things or good things, it really means all things.

When things happen which seem to be disastrous or extremely challenging, I know that if I trust the Lord with all my heart, and I do not rely on my own understanding of the situation, God will work it out for me. I can trust the Lord and rely on Him. I do not have to worry because all things happen for good to those who love the Lord. It gives me tremendous peace of mind to know that God is taking care of me. He has seen fit to put me on this earth and get me through the world better than I can with my own understanding and efforts at trying to analyze the situation. I know God will work it out. All I need to do is trust God with all my heart and keep working in health, happiness, and faith.

STEP 4. *Use the power of love*

Expressing love is the most important factor in expressing spirituality. The Bible says in First Corinthians Chapter 13, "If I have the gift of prophecy and can fathom all mysteries and all knowledge, and if I have a faith that can move mountains, but have not love, I am nothing. If I give all I possess to the poor and surrender my body to the flames, but have not love, I gain nothing. Love is patient, love is kind. It does not envy, it does not boast, it is not proud. It is not rude, it is not self-seeking, it is not easily angered, it keeps no record of wrongs. Love does not delight in evil but rejoices with the truth. It always protects, always trusts, always hopes, always perseveres. Love never fails."

We all need to have love in our lives. Love is the most important factor between family members, friends, business associates, customers—everyone. We are all God's children. We are all human beings. We need to learn to love each other.

When we love another human being unconditionally, something wonderful happens—we get love back. One of the key principles of life is that whatever you sow, so shall you reap, but multiplied a hundred times. When you plant a tomato seed, you get a bush of tomatoes—a tomato plant that has dozens of tomatoes on it, each of which has dozens of seeds. The law of nature always gives back more than it receives. And really, it is the same for human beings. If we feel that we are lacking, it is only because we are not giving that thing which we are lacking. We all need and want love, but in order to receive love we must first give.

The principle of reaping what you sow (or of karma) applies to anything that we want. It does require faith and trust. A farmer will not go out and dig up the seed to see if it is growing. The same is true in the human process. If you disturb the process, or worry, you block the vital energy that is creating what you desire, and you have to start all over again. The farmer doesn't go into his house and sit in a rocking chair and stare out the window at the soil and worry because he hasn't seen anything happen yet. He goes about his business. He comes back one day, and suddenly, the seeds are all up. And he has hundreds and hundreds more seeds than he planted. And that's the way life is. Life works on exactly the same principles. To make a better life for ourselves and a better world, all we need to do is plant more seeds of love in the hearts of all with whom we come into contact.

Before we can love others, we must first learn to love and accept ourselves. This is a tough challenge for most people because we fail to realize that we are a part of God. If we can accept ourselves, it is much easier to accept others because, as we look at ourselves, we are looking at everyone else. Often when people do not accept others or belittle them, it is because they are trying to raise themselves up to a superior level by using others as a stepping stone. As these people with low levels of self-love and acceptance tear down others, they feel they are building themselves up. In actuality, however, they are undermining their own self-esteem and self-acceptance.

When a person criticizes or judges other people harshly, such thoughts and feelings are really tearing down his or her own health.

To paraphrase St. Matthew Chapter 7, we should not judge others. Instead of looking for the faults in other people, we should examine our own and cast them out. Our focus should be on bringing good from ourselves and others.

Through self-acceptance and self-love, we become more accepting and loving of others. Expressing spirituality to others means looking past or through human frailties and imperfections and seeing that inside each person is a spirit that is perfect and godlike. Sometimes it may be hard to look through superficial human qualities, but, for your health and that of others, try to see the true spiritual beings within rather than focus on the shortcomings of human behavior.

In Chapter 3, Key #3—Positive Relationships, we will discuss further the importance of love in raising human health.

STEP 5. *Become a servant of others*

The Bible clearly shows us that the servant will be the greatest among us. I think when we humble ourselves and serve others, that is where we begin our greatest reward. And we are the ones who actually receive. One of my favorite inspirational teachers, Zig Ziglar, author of *See You at the Top* and *Top Performance*, has a very powerful philosophy. Zig teaches that we can have everything we want in life if we simply help enough people get what they want. Basically, what Zig is reinforcing is the principle of being a servant of others.

I have incorporated the principle of servitude and Zig's philosophy not only in my personal life, but also in the core philosophy at Enzymatic Therapy. The principle works. Our goal is not to sell products. Our goal is not to make money. Instead, our goal is to help people. We help people get what they want. If people do not get what they want from one of our products, we offer a complete 100% PLUS money-back guarantee. We also do our best to educate and teach people the value of good nutrition and good health. We are not concerned about the rewards for our service; we have trust and faith in God that if we follow the guidelines He has laid down for us, we will be rewarded.

In my personal life, I have found that when I help others, it makes me feel better about myself. Think about a time in your life when you helped a friend or, better yet, a stranger. How did it make you feel when you gave of yourself freely? When I have asked people the question, "Can you describe a time in your life when you felt the best about yourself?" invariably, they will describe a time when they gave of themselves to help (serve) another human being. It is a tremendous feeling. Somehow, through a mechanism which I don't quite understand, we just tend to feel fantastic. Maybe this feeling is what God meant when He said that the servant would be the greatest of all and would be exalted.

STEP 6. *Tithe*

Tithing is probably one of the most misunderstood and most overlooked principles of life. Tithing, according to the Bible, is giving 10% of our income to God's work. Where we tithe can be an individual choice, but our tithes should really go directly to God's work, so we must choose carefully. Tithes should probably go where we get most of our spiritual support, such as our church. We can also tithe directly to the poor. The Bible says in Psalms 41:1-3, "God blesses those who are kind to the poor. He helps them out of their troubles. He protects them and keeps them alive; He publicly honors them and destroys the power of their enemies. He nurses them when they are sick, and soothes their pains and worries."

Search out and determine a beneficiary for your tithe. I believe that if everybody who reads this book would tithe, their lives would be greatly enhanced. It is unbelievable what tithing can do. I have had the privilege of talking to some people who are now tithing 90% of their income, because the remaining 5 to 10% of their income is as much as most people wish they could make in a lifetime.

The only place in the Bible where God says, "Test Me, and see if I am not telling you the truth," is in Malachi Chapter 3. It reads:

> "Return to me, and I will return to you," says the Lord Almighty.
> But you ask, "How are we to return?"
> "Will a man rob God? Yet you rob me."
> But you ask, "How do we rob you?"
> "In tithes and offerings. You are under a curse—the whole nation of you—because you are robbing me. Bring the whole tithe into the storehouse, that there may be food in my house. Test me in this," says the Lord Almighty, "and see if I will not throw open the floodgates of heaven and pour out so much blessing that you will not have enough room for it."

I believe in the power of these words and the power of tithing. I have used tithing throughout my life. My company tithes, my children tithe, and my employees tithe because tithing is a principle that works. I believe that if somebody wants to be healthy and successful, without any other beliefs attached, they must tithe. Tithe because God will bless you. How can you pass up this opportunity?

STEP 7. *Attend church regularly*

The last step in achieving spirituality is attending church. While some may consider this step the sole factor in defining a person's spirituality, I do not use it as a yardstick to measure a person's spirituality. And yet, I consider it important.

A church brings people together in a very special way. It allows people to express their spirituality, pray together, and extend love to one another. And, according to many studies, people who attend church regularly have better health.

In a recent survey of 1,473 people, a research team led by Purdue University psychologist Kenneth Ferraro found that only 59 who went to church reported ill health compared to 133 who did not. Also, 530 of the "weekly attenders" reported excellent health, compared to only 383 of the "never attenders."

For the study, Dr. Ferraro looked at three aspects: frequency of attendance at church or synagogue; the experiential aspect, or sense of feeling close to God; and the specific creed or beliefs. Of these three factors, only active participation was found to make a big difference, with higher participation linked to better health. The big question is why? The researchers offered four possible explanations:

1. People who attend church regularly tend to avoid health-destructive behaviors such as smoking and using drugs or alcohol.
2. Religious activity provides a social network for coping and support that is quite different from our secular network.
3. Faith provides a special meaning and value system to help us make sense of the world and our lives.
4. Religious practice helps us cope with physical suffering and gives us hope.

I believe one of the big reasons church-going people are healthier is that they are regularly reminded of important values. Rather than material possessions, religion values human traits we all can admire: honesty, compassion, loyalty, friendship, fellowship, and love.

CHAPTER TWO

KEY #2—POSITIVE ATTITUDE

STEP 1.
Become an optimist

STEP 2.
Practice positive self-talk

STEP 3.
Ask better questions

STEP 4.
Employ positive affirmations

STEP 5.
Set positive goals

STEP 6.
Use positive visualization

STEP 7.
Read or listen to positive messages

KEY #2—POSITIVE ATTITUDE

More and more evidence clearly demonstrates that what we think and feel has a tremendous effect on the way our body functions. The most important factor in maintaining or attaining health is a consistent "positive mental attitude." Researchers in the medical and psychological fields are demonstrating that our level of optimism is a major determining factor in our level of wellness.

The steps described in this chapter are necessary not only for achieving vibrant health, but also for achieving a life full of passion, happiness, joy, and fun. View your attitude as an entity like the human body. It needs nourishment, care, and conditioning. For most people, a positive attitude doesn't happen all at once. It happens by degrees, subtle changes accumulating one by one. Would you be in good physical condition if you exercised only once? No. It takes conditioning. The same is true for your attitude.

Life is full of events beyond our control. However, while we do not have any control over these events, we do have control over our response to them. Our attitude determines how we view and respond to the challenges of life. You will be much happier, healthier, and more successful if you can adopt a positive mental attitude rather than a pessimistic view.

STEP 1. *Become an optimist*

The first step in developing a positive mental attitude is to become an optimist. This shouldn't be too hard. According to Martin Seligman, Ph.D., author of *Learned Optimism* and one the world's leading authorities on optimism, we are, by nature, optimists. Optimism is a necessary step towards achieving health as well as our goals in life. Research is revealing that optimism not only prevents disease, but also is a vital ally in the healing process. Conversely, a pessimistic attitude can seriously erode our health.

Several research studies indicate that chronically angry, suspicious, and mistrustful people are twice as likely to have coronary artery blockages. And during periods of grief, the T cells—important white blood cells which fight against infection and cancer—do not multiply as quickly.

What distinguishes an optimist from a pessimist is the way that each explains both good and bad events. Dr. Seligman has developed a simple test to determine your level of optimism. Try his test and evaluate your outlook.

Are you an optimist?

To determine whether you are an optimist, answer the following questions. Take as much time as you need. There are no right or wrong answers. It is important that you take the test before you read the interpretation. Read the description of each situation and vividly imagine it happening to you. Choose the response that most applies to you by circling either A or B. Ignore the letter and number codes for now; they will be explained later.

Test your optimism

1. The project you are in charge of is a great success.

	PsG
A. *I kept a close watch over everyone's work.*	1
B. *Everyone devoted a lot of time and energy to it.*	0

2. You and your spouse (boyfriend/girlfriend) make up after a fight.

	PmG
A. *I forgave him/her.*	0
B. *I'm usually forgiving.*	1

3. You get lost driving to a friend's house.

	PsB
A. *I missed a turn.*	1
B. *My friend gave me bad directions.*	0

4. Your spouse (boyfriend/girlfriend) surprises you with a gift.

	PsG
A. *He/she just got a raise at work.*	0
B. *I took him/her out to a special dinner the night before.*	1

5. You forgot your spouse's (boyfriend's/girlfriend's) birthday.

	PmB
A. *I'm not good at remembering birthdays.*	1
B. *I was preoccupied with other things.*	0

6. You get a flower from a secret admirer.

	PvG
A. *I am attractive to him/her.*	0
B. *I am a popular person.*	1

7. You run for a community office position and you win.

	PvG
A. *I devote a lot of time and energy to campaigning.*	0
B. *I work very hard at everything I do.*	1

8. You miss an important engagement.

	PvB
A. *Sometimes my memory fails me.*	1
B. *I sometimes forget to check my appointment book.*	0

9. You run for a community office position and you lose.

	PsB
A. *I didn't campaign hard enough.*	1
B. *The person who won knew more people.*	0

10. You host a successful dinner.

	PmG
A. *I was particularly charming that night.*	0
B. *I am a good host.*	1

11. You stop a crime by calling the police.

	PsG
A. *A strange noise caught my attention.*	0
B. *I was alert that day.*	1

12. You were extremely healthy all year.

	PsG
A. *Few people around me were sick, so I wasn't exposed.*	0
B. *I made sure I ate well and got enough rest.*	1

13. You owe the library ten dollars for an overdue book.

	PmB
A. *When I am really involved in what I am reading, I often forget when it's due.*	1
B. *I was so involved in writing the report that I forgot to return the book.*	0

14. Your stocks make you a lot of money.

	PmG
A. *My broker decided to take on something new.*	0
B. *My broker is a top-notch investor.*	1

15. You win an athletic contest.

                                                            PmG

    A. I was feeling unbeatable.   0

    B. I train hard.   1

16. You fail an important examination.

                                                            PvB

    A. I wasn't as smart as the other people taking the exam.   1

    B. I didn't prepare for it well.   0

17. You prepared a special meal for a friend and
he/she barely touched the food.

                                                            PvB

    A. I wasn't a good cook.   1

    B. I made the meal in a rush.   0

18. You lose a sporting event for which you have
been training for a long time.

                                                            PvB

    A. I'm not very athletic.   1

    B. I'm not good at that sport.   0

19. Your car runs out of gas on a dark street late at night.

                                                            PsB

    A. I didn't check to see how much gas was in the tank.   1

    B. The gas gauge was broken.   0

20. You lose your temper with a friend.

                                                            PmB

    A. He/she is always nagging me.   1

    B. He/she was in a hostile mood.   0

21. You are penalized for not returning your income-tax
forms on time.

                                                            PmB

    A. I always put off doing my taxes.   1

    B. I was lazy about getting my taxes done this year.   0

22. You ask a person out on a date and he/she says no.

                                                            PvB

    A. I was a wreck that day.   1

    B. I got tongue-tied when I asked him/her on the date.   0

23. A game-show host picks you out of the audience to
participate in the show.

                                                            PsG

    A. I was sitting in the right seat.   0

    B. I looked the most enthusiastic.   1

24. You are frequently asked to dance at a party.

                                                                   PmG

    A. I am outgoing at parties.   1
    B. I was in perfect form that night.   0

25. You buy your spouse (boyfriend/girlfriend) a gift and he/she doesn't like it.

        PsB

    A. I don't put enough thought into things like that.   1
    B. He/she has very picky tastes.   0

26. You do exceptionally well in a job interview.

    PmG

    A. I felt extremely confident during the interview.   0
    B. I interview well.   1

27. You tell a joke and everyone laughs.

    PsG

    A. The joke was funny.   0
    B. My timing was perfect.   1

28. Your boss gives you too little time in which to finish a project, but you get it finished anyway.

    PvG

    A. I am good at my job.   0
    B. I am an efficient person.   1

29. You've been feeling run-down lately.

    PmB

    A. I never get a chance to relax.   1
    B. I was exceptionally busy this week.   0

30. You ask someone to dance and he/she says no.

    PsB

    A. I am not a good enough dancer.   1
    B. He/she doesn't like to dance.   0

31. You save a person from choking to death.

    PvG

    A. I know a technique to stop someone from choking.   0
    B. I know what to do in crisis situations.   1

32. Your romantic partner wants to cool things off for a while.

    PvB

    A. I'm too self-centered.   1
    B. I don't spend enough time with him/her.   0

33. A friend says something that hurts your feelings.

                                                 PmB

    A. *She always blurts things out without thinking*
       of others.   1
    B. *My friend was in a bad mood and took it out on me.*   0

34. Your employer comes to you for advice.

                                                 PvG

    A. *I am an expert in the area about which I was asked.*   0
    B. *I'm good at giving useful advice.*   1

35. A friend thanks you for helping him/her get through a bad time.

                                                 PvG

    A. *I enjoy helping him/her through tough times.*   0
    B. *I care about people.*   1

36. You have a wonderful time at a party.

                                               PsG

    A. *Everyone was friendly.*   0
    B. *I was friendly.*   1

37. Your doctor tells you that you are in good physical shape.

                                             PvG

    A. *I make sure I exercise frequently.*   0
    B. *I am very health-conscious.*   1

38. Your spouse (boyfriend/girlfriend) takes you away for a romantic weekend.

                                             PmG

    A. *He/she needed to get away for a few days.*   0
    B. *He/she likes to explore new areas.*   1

39. Your doctor tells you that you eat too much sugar.

                                             PsB

    A. *I don't pay much attention to my diet.*   1
    B. *You can't avoid sugar, it's in everything.*   0

40. You are asked to head an important project.

                                             PmG

    A. *I just successfully completed a similar project.*   0
    B. *I am a good supervisor.*   1

41. You and your spouse (boyfriend/girlfriend) have been fighting a great deal.

                                             PsB

    A. *I have been feeling cranky and pressured lately.*   1
    B. *He/she has been hostile lately.*   0

42. You fall down a great deal while skiing.

	PmB
A. Skiing is difficult.	1
B. The trails were icy.	0

43. You win a prestigious award.

	PvG
A. I solved an important problem.	0
B. I was the best employee.	1

44. Your stocks are at an all-time low.

	PvB
A. I didn't know much about the business climate at the time.	1
B. I made a poor choice of stocks.	0

45. You win the lottery.

	PsG
A. It was pure chance.	0
B. I picked the right numbers.	1

46. You gain weight over the holidays and you can't lose it.

	PmB
A. Diets don't work in the long run.	1
B. The diet I tried didn't work.	0

47. You are in the hospital and few people come to visit.

	PsB
A. I'm irritable when I am sick.	1
B. My friends are negligent about things like that.	0

48. They won't honor your credit card at a store.

	PvB
A. I sometimes overestimate how much money I have.	1
B. I sometimes forget to pay my credit card bill.	0

Scoring Key

PmB _____	PmG _____
PvB _____	PvG _____

HoB _____

PsB _____	PsG _____
Total B _____	Total G _____

G-B _____

Interpreting your test

The test results will give you a clue as to your explanatory style. In other words, the results will tell you how you explain things to yourself. It will show you your habitual way of thinking. Again, remember, there are no right or wrong answers.

Your explanatory style is composed of three crucial dimensions: permanence, pervasiveness, and personalization. Each dimension, plus a couple of others, will be scored from your test.

Permanence

When pessimists are faced with challenges or bad events, they view these events as being permanent. In contrast, people who are optimists tend to view the challenges or bad events as temporary. Here are some statements that reflect some subtle differences:

Pessimistic (Permanent)	Optimistic (Temporary)
"My boss is always a jerk."	"My boss is in a bad mood today."
"You never listen."	"You are not listening."
"I'm an unlucky person."	"This event was unfortunate."

To determine how you view bad events, look at the eight items coded PmB (for Permanent Bad): 5, 13, 20, 21, 29, 33, 42, and 46. Each one followed by a 0 is optimistic, while each one followed by a 1 is pessimistic. Total the numbers at the right-hand margin of the questions coded PmB and write the total on the PmB line on the scoring key.

If you totaled 0 or 1, you are very optimistic in this dimension; 2 or 3 is a moderately optimistic score; 4 is average; 5 or 6 is pessimistic; a 7 or 8 is extremely pessimistic.

Now let's take a look at the difference in explanatory style between pessimists and optimists when a positive event occurs in their lives. It's just the opposite of what happened with a bad event. Pessimists view positive events as temporary while optimists view them as permanent. Here again are some subtle differences in how pessimists and optimists might communicate their good fortune:

Pessimistic (Temporary)	Optimistic (Permanent)
"I'm lucky for once."	"I'm such a lucky person."
"My opponent was off today."	"I am getting better every day."
"I tried hard today."	"I always give my best."

Now total all the questions coded PmG (for Permanent Good): 2, 10, 14, 15, 24, 26, 38, and 40. Write the total on the line in the scoring key marked PmG.

If you totaled 7 or 8, you are very optimistic in this dimension; 6 is a moderately optimistic score; 4 or 5 is average; 3 is pessimistic; a 0, 1 or 2 is extremely pessimistic.

Are you starting to see a pattern? If you are scoring as a pessimist, you may want to learn how to be more optimistic. Your anxiety may be due to your belief that bad things are always going to happen, while good things are only a fluke.

Pervasiveness

Pervasiveness is the tendency to describe things in universals (everyone, always, never, etc.) versus specifics (a specific individual, a specific time, etc.). Pessimists tend to describe things in universals while optimists describe things in specifics.

Pessimist (Universal)	*Optimist (Specific)*
"All lawyers are jerks."	"My attorney was a jerk."
"He is repulsive."	"He is repulsive to me."
"Instruction manuals are worthless."	"This instruction manual is worthless."

Total your score for the questions coded PvB (for Pervasive Bad): 8, 16, 17, 18, 22, 32, 44, and 48. Write the total on the PvB line.

If you totaled 0 or 1, you are very optimistic in this dimension; 2 or 3 is a moderately optimistic score; 4 is average; 5 or 6 is pessimistic; a 7 or 8 is extremely pessimistic.

Now let's look at the level of pervasiveness of good events. Optimists tend to view good events as universal, while pessimists view them as specific. Again, it's just the opposite of how each views a bad event.

Total your score for the questions coded PvG (for Pervasive Good): 6, 7, 28, 31, 34, 35, 37, and 43. Write the total on the line labeled PvG.

If you totaled 7 or 8, you are very optimistic in this dimension; 6 is a moderately optimistic score; 4 or 5 is average; 3 is pessimistic; a 0, 1 or 2 is extremely pessimistic.

Hope

Our level of hope or hopelessness is determined by our combined level of permanence and pervasiveness. Your level of hope may be the most significant score for this test. Take your PvB and add it to your PmB score. This is your hope score.

If it is 0, 1, or 2, you are extraordinarily hopeful; 3, 4, 5, or 6 is a moderately hopeful score; 7 or 8 is average; 9, 10, or 11 is moderately hopeless; and 12, 13, 14, 15, or 16 is severely hopeless.

People who make permanent and universal explanations for their troubles tend to suffer from stress, anxiety, and depression. When things go bad, they collapse. According to Dr. Seligman, no other score is as important as your hope score.

Personalization

The final aspect of explanatory style is personalization. When bad things happen, we can either assume all the blame ourselves (internalize) and lower our self-esteem as a consequence, or we can put some of the blame on things beyond our control (externalize). Although it may not be right to deny any personal responsibility, people who tend to externalize some of the blame for bad events have higher self-esteem and are more optimistic.

Total your score for the questions coded PsB (for Personalization Bad): 3, 9, 19, 25, 30, 39, 41, and 47. Write the total on the PsB line.

A score of 0 or 1 indicates very high self-esteem and optimism; 2 or 3 indicates moderate self-esteem; 4 is average; 5 or 6 indicates moderately low self-esteem; and 7 or 8 indicates very low self-esteem.

Now let's take a look at personalization and good events. Again, just the exact opposite interpretation occurs compared to bad events. When good things happen, the person with high self-esteem internalizes while the person with low self-esteem externalizes.

Total your score for the questions coded PsG (for Personalization Good): 1, 4, 11, 12, 23, 27, 36, and 45. Write your total on the line marked PsG on the scoring key.

If you totaled 7 or 8, you are very optimistic in this dimension; 6 is a moderately optimistic score; 4 or 5 is average; 3 is pessimistic; a 0, 1 or 2 is extremely pessimistic.

Your overall scores

To compute your overall scores, first add the three Bs (PmB + PvB + PsB). This is your B (bad event) score. Do the same for all of the Gs (PmG + PvG + PsG). This is your G (good event) score. Subtract B from G; this is your overall score.

If your B score is from 3 to 6, you are marvelously optimistic when bad events occur; 10 or 11 is average; 12 to 14 is pessimistic; anything above 14 is extremely pessimistic.

If your G score is 19 or above, you are extremely optimistic in your thoughts about good events; 14 to 16 is average; 11 to 13 indicates pessimism; and a score of 10 or less indicates great pessimism.

If your overall score (G minus B) is above 8, you are very optimistic across the board; if it's from 6 to 8 you are moderately optimistic; 3 to 5 is average; 1 or 2 is pessimistic; and a score of zero or below is very pessimistic.

Optimism and health

Optimists have been shown to possess greater health. Consider the findings of researcher Christopher Peterson, Ph.D., professor of psychology at the University of Michigan. He and his colleagues analyzed data from a 35-year research project known as the Harvard Study of Adult Development. The 268 men in the study were drawn from the Harvard classes of 1942 and 1944. They were chosen on the basis of their academic success, sound physical and psychological health, and high level of independence and accomplishment as determined by college deans.

Test subjects' optimism scores were compared with their health ratings as determined by doctors. They underwent physical exams at age 25 and every five years afterward. It's no surprise that those who scored higher for optimism remained healthier later in life than the men who were more pessimistic.

Naturally, optimistic people are more inclined to look after their own health. They are more likely to work out, eat a balanced diet, and get regular medical checkups. Optimists respond to illness actively, consulting their doctor promptly and following a responsible treatment plan.

Learning optimism

It is important to learn how to be optimistic if you are a pessimist. Why? Again, studies have shown that optimists are healthier, happier, and enjoy life at a much higher level than pessimists. Learning to be optimistic means that you need to get in the habit of thinking with a positive attitude. If you are pessimistic, it is only because you habitually think in a negative framework.

Is it possible to learn optimism? More psychologists are saying yes. Cognitive therapy, originally developed by psychiatrist Aaron T. Beck and psychologist Albert Ellis, is based on the premise that our thoughts control our feelings. In other words, if we can adopt more positive habits of thought, we can make ourselves feel better.

The Complete Guide to Your Emotions & Your Health, by Emrika Padus and the editors of *Prevention* magazine, explains that negative thinking is a learned response. Six common pessimistic distortions are exaggerating, ignoring the positive, personalizing, either/or thinking, over-generalizing, and jumping to conclusions. Gary Emery, Ph.D., author of *A New Beginning*, writes, "The chief characteristic of negative thoughts is that they're generally wrong."

To "reprogram" your thinking, *The Complete Guide* suggests that you become aware of the unfocused negative thoughts that leap into your mind uninvited. Write them down. Then respond to them with more realistic, constructive, and adaptive thinking.

Another book, *Feeling Good*, by David Burns, offers the following suggestions for becoming more optimistic:

- Choose an area of your life in which you want to begin thinking and acting more optimistically.
- Become aware of your thoughts and beliefs in this area.
- Ask yourself how realistic these beliefs are.
- Set modest and immediate goals for changing your habits of thinking.
- As you make those changes successfully, reward yourself.
- Seek out the company of optimistic people.
- Be playful about your venture into optimism.
- Remember that optimism is healthy, in part, because it leads to action.
- Ask your friends and family members to help you.
- Make some positive changes in your lifestyle.
- Be flexible. Use these suggestions in whatever way seems best to you. Don't let setbacks or delays discourage you.

Cognitive thinking is a skill-building process. With time, effort, and commitment, anyone can replace the habit of negative thinking with a new habit of more constructive, positive thinking. And that's a vital step toward better health.

STEP 2. *Practice positive self-talk*

To be truly healthy, we must have positive self-talk. By self-talk, I am referring to the type of language used by your brain. Self-talk is a powerful tool in creating a positive attitude.

Self-talk plugs directly into our subconscious which either tells us how we are going to feel or starts the process of creating a "self-fulfilling prophecy." For example, how do you usually respond when somebody says, "How are you?" I believe that your routine answer to this question goes a long way in determining your dominant emotional and physical state. If your answer is "not too bad," then that becomes your dominant state. If your answer is "O.K.," then that becomes your dominant state.

When people ask me how I am, I always say something like "super," "great," "fantastic," "phenomenal," or, on occasion, "ecstatic." Even though I may not feel great that day, in time, if I continue to say how I want to feel, then that will become my dominant state. I know this may sound kind of strange, but all I can say is try it for yourself. It's fun to watch how people respond. Usually they will say, "Wow, what is going on in your life that is so fantastic?" Your response to this question is to focus on all of the positive things in your life which, in turn, increases your positive mental attitude and attracts even more things to be thankful for.

Some people might have a hard time believing in the power of positive self-talk, but if they take the opportunity to use it, I know it can dramatically improve the quality of their life. Two powerful tools for creating positive self-talk are questions and affirmations (discussed next).

STEP 3. *Ask better questions*

One of the most powerful tools I have found for improving the quality of my self-talk and the quality of my life is a series of questions originally given to me by Anthony Robbins, author of the bestsellers, *Unlimited Power* and *Awaken the Giant Within*. According to Tony, the quality of your life is equal to the quality of the questions you habitually ask yourself. Tony's statement is based on his belief that whatever question you ask your brain, is the question your brain will answer.

Let's look at the following example: An individual is met with a particular challenge or problem. He or she can ask a number of questions in this situation. Questions many people ask in such circumstances include: "Why does this always happen to me?" Or, "Why am I always so stupid?" Do they get answers to these questions? Do the answers build self-esteem? Does the problem keep reappearing? What would be a higher quality question? How about: "This is a very interesting situation. What do I need to learn from this situation so it never happens again?" Or, "What can I do to make this situation better?"

In another example, let's look at an individual who suffers from depression. What are some questions he or she might ask which may not be helping the situation? How about: "Why am I always so depressed?" "Why do things always seem to go wrong for me?" "Why am I doomed to be so unhappy?"

What are some better questions they may want to ask themselves? How about: "What do I need to do to gain more enjoyment and happiness in my life?" "What do I need to commit to in order to have more happiness and energy in my life?" After they have answered these questions, they could ask themselves this one: "If I had happiness and high energy levels right now, what would it feel like?"

You will be amazed at how powerful questions can be in your life. When the mind is searching for answers to these questions, it is reprogramming your subconscious into believing you have an abundance of energy. Unless there is a physiological reason for the chronic fatigue, it won't take long before your subconscious believes.

Regardless of the situation, asking better questions is bound to improve your attitude. If you want to have a better life, simply ask better questions. It sounds simple because it is. If you want more energy, excitement, and happiness in your life, ask yourself the following questions on a consistent basis.

The Morning Questions
1. What am I most happy about in my life right now?
   Why does that make me happy?
   How does that make me feel?
2. What am I most excited about in my life right now?
   Why does that make me excited?
   How does that make me feel?

3. What am I most grateful for in my life right now?
   Why does that make me grateful?
   How does that make me feel?
4. What am I enjoying most about my life right now?
   What about that do I enjoy?
   How does that make me feel?
5. What am I committed to in my life right now?
   Why am I committed to that?
   How does that make me feel?
6. Who do I love? (Starting close and moving out)
   Who loves me?
8. What must I do today to achieve my long-term goal?

The Evening Questions

1. What have I given today?
   In what ways have I been a giver today?
2. What did I learn today?
3. What did I do today to reach my long-term goal?
4. In what ways was today a perfect day?
5. Repeat morning questions

The Problem or Challenge Questions

1. What is right/great about this problem?
2. What is not perfect yet?
3. What am I willing to do to make it the way I want it
   to be?
4. How can I enjoy doing the things necessary to
   make it the way I want it to be?

STEP 4. *Employ positive affirmations*

An affirmation is a positive statement. Affirmations can make imprints on the subconscious mind to create a healthy, positive self-image. In addition, affirmations can actually fuel the changes you desire. I use certain phrases and sentences as affirmations each day. Some of my favorites are:

- I can do all things through Christ who gives me
  the strength.
- I feel healthy. I feel great. I feel terrific.
- Money flows through me freely for the good of
  others.

- Love flows through me in avalanches of abundance.

Here are some very simple guidelines for creating your own affirmations.

1. Always phrase an affirmation in the present tense. Imagine that it has already come to pass.
2. Always phrase the affirmation as a positive statement. Avoid the words "not" or "never."
3. Do your best to totally identify with the positive feelings that are generated by the affirmation.
4. Keep the affirmation short and simple but full of feeling. Be creative.
5. Imagine yourself really experiencing what you are affirming.
6. Make the affirmation personal to you and full of meaning.

Using these guidelines and examples, write down five affirmations that apply to you. State these affirmations aloud while you are taking your shower, driving, or when you are praying.

STEP 5. *Set positive goals*

Learning to set goals in a positive way is another powerful method for building a positive attitude and raising self-esteem. Goals can be used to create a "success cycle." Achieving goals helps you feel better about yourself, and the better you feel about yourself, the more likely you will achieve your goals. Here are some guidelines to use when setting goals.

1. State the goal in positive terms; avoid any negative words in your goal statement. For example, it is better to say "I enjoy eating healthy, low-calorie, nutritious foods" than "I will not eat sugar, candy, ice cream, and other fattening foods." Remember, always state the goal in positive terms, and avoid any negative words in the goal statement.

2. Make your goal attainable and realistic. Again, you can use goals to create a success cycle and positive self-image. Little things add up to make a major difference in the way you feel about yourself.

3. Be specific. The more clearly your goal is defined, the more likely you are to reach it. For example, if you want to lose weight, what is the weight you desire? What body fat percentage or measurements do you desire? Clearly define just what you want to achieve.

4. State the goal in the present tense, not the future tense. In order to reach your goal, you have to believe you have already attained it. You must literally program yourself to achieve the goal. See and feel yourself having already achieved the goal and success will be yours. Remember,always state your goal in the present tense.

Any voyage begins with one step and is followed by many other steps. Remember to set short-term goals which can be used to help you achieve your long-term goals. Get in the habit of asking yourself the following question each morning and evening: What must I do today to achieve my long-term goal?

STEP 6. *Use positive visualization*

Positive visualization or imagery is another powerful tool for creating health, happiness, and success. I believe that we have to be able to see our lives the way we want them to be before it happens.

A number of excellent books can help inspire you with accounts of the power of positive visualization. One of the first books I read on this subject was Maxwell Maltz's now classic work, *Psycho-Cybernetics*. Another excellent book is Dr. Wayne Dyer's *You'll See It When You Believe It*.

Most of the initial research on the power of visualization focused on enhancing physical performance. For example, in *Psycho-Cybernetics*, Maltz recounts an experiment comparing the effect of visualization versus physical practice in improving basketball free throw shooting.

One group of students actually practiced shooting free throws for twenty minutes each day for twenty days and were scored on the first and last day. A second group was scored on the first and last days, but engaged in no sort of practice in between. A third group was scored on the first and last days, but spent twenty minutes on each of the intervening days visualizing shooting free throws successfully.

The results? Visualization was just as effective as actual physical practice. The first group improved 24%, the second group showed no improvement, and the third group improved 23%.

The power of positive visualization is discussed extensively in *Peak Performance* by Dr. Charles Garfield, a psychologist who has done extensive research on peak performance, both in business and athletics. While working with the NASA program, Dr. Garfield became fascinated with the power of visualization as he watched astronauts rehearse scenes over and over in their heads, so they would be prepared when they went into space. Although he had a doctorate in mathematics, he decided to go back to school and get a Ph.D. in the field of psychology. His focus was to better understand the characteristics of successful people.

One of Dr. Garfield's key findings is that almost all world-class athletes and other peak performers employ positive visualization. They see their goal, they feel it, and identify with it so strongly emotionally that they actually experience it before they do it. It all begins in the mind's eye.

You can use visualization in all areas of your life, but especially for your health. In fact, some of the most promising research on the power of visualization involves enhancing the immune system in the treatment of cancer. Much of the pioneering work in this field has been conducted at the Simonton Research Center in Dallas, Texas, under the supervision of Carl Simonton, M.D. Along with standard medical treatment, Dr. Simonton teaches patients how to imagine white blood cells as little Pac-Men digesting and destroying tumors. Dr. Simonton's techniques are described in his book, *Getting Well Again*.

Dr. Simonton and others are showing that positive visualization is proving to be very powerful medicine. For example, a study conducted at Yale University demonstrated that patients suffering from severe depression were helped considerably by simply imagining scenes in which they were praised by people they admired. Be creative and have fun with positive visualizations, and you will soon find yourself living your dreams.

To help get you started, here is an excellent visualization script excerpted from *Rituals of Healing—Using Imagery for Health and Wellness* by Jeanne Acterberg, Barbara Dossey, and Leslie Kolkmeier. Use it to promote overall healing and general well-being.

Before you begin your imagery journey, find a quiet, comfortable place, and give yourself permission to spend fifteen or twenty minutes taking care of yourself. Lie down, or sit with your back and neck completely supported. Allow your chair, or bed, or wherever you are to hold you. Let tension melt away as you bring your attention to your breath, listening to, feeling the in breath, the out breath...[Pause for one minute.] Take a mental journey now, through your body, beginning at the bottom of your feet. Move your attention slowly to the top of your head, letting go of any tightness or restriction you find. [Pause for one or two minutes, or guide yourself through your muscle groups.]

Your mind has just moved through your body, connecting with it, giving it attention, soothing the tense, tired places. Now let your mind move to a still point. Some people find this still point deep within, a place of pure peace and calm, a place of quiet knowing. Let the words "still point" fill your mind, chasing out other thoughts and concerns. Breathe yourself into this quiet place. Quietly, gently find the stillness. [Pause one minute.]

Sit comfortably, with your back straight but relaxed. Focus on your breath and inhale and exhale three times. Then, slowly, begin to inhale.

As you feel the air moving in through your nose and down the back of your throat into your lungs, hear yourself saying, way in the back of your mind..."One."...Feel the air moving back out...As the next breath begins to fill your lungs, hear yourself saying, deep inside of yourself..."Two."...Feel the air moving back out...With the next breath in, hear yourself saying, deep inside of yourself..."Three."...Feel the air moving back out...With the next breath in, hear yourself saying, deep inside of yourself..."Four."...Feel the air moving back out...Repeat this cycle as many times as you wish, counting one to four with your breaths.

With each breath in...feel your diaphragm moving down toward your feet...and your lower abdomen beginning to expand...With each breath out...as your abdomen relaxes...feel the muscles in your neck and shoulders drifting down with gravity...and relaxing even more deeply.

Imagine your body is made of a beautiful, clear, crystalline material...Each time you breathe in, imagine your breath is a healing, colored mist...any color that comes to mind...Feel the healing mist entering your body through the top of your head and drifting slowly down inside your crystal-clear body...See and feel that mist beginning to fill you with relaxation and calm... Each breath slowly fills your crystal body with peace and healing...Continue to see yourself filling with color until your body is completely full of relaxation.

With the next breath in, say to yourself, "I am breathing..." As you breathe out, say to yourself, "warmth into my feet."...With the next breath in, say to yourself, "I am breathing..." As you breathe out, say to yourself, "warmth into my legs."...Continue in this manner, breathing warmth into all parts of your body...Gradually come back to full awareness of the room and notice your calmness and relaxation.

This relaxation technique is phenomenally effective for dealing with stress. It feels fantastic to let go of all the pressures of modern living. I use this technique often not only for visualization exercises, but also for magnifying prayer and meditation.

Realizing that our actions, feelings, and behavior are the results of our internal images gives us a powerful tool for gaining new skills, success, greater happiness, and better health.

STEP 7. *Read or listen to positive messages*

Achieving a positive mental attitude is very similar to achieving a highly conditioned physical body. Just like the physical body, we must exercise and condition our attitude. All of the steps discussed in this chapter are important in this effort. The final step, reading or listening to positive messages, is one that helps me continually renew my motivation and inspiration. While driving, exercising, cooking or doing chores around the house, I take advantage of tapes that nourish my attitude with good, positive, inspirational information. Before going to sleep, I always take a few minutes to read something that fills my mind with positive thoughts.

Here are some of the authors and books (in alphabetical order by author) that have inspired me the most. Most of these authors also have tapes available. A good resource for tapes is the Nightingale-Conant company (1-800-525-9000).

Buscaglia, Leo
  Living, Loving, and Learning
  Loving Each Other

Carnegie, Dale
  How to Win Friends & Influence People

Covey, Stephen R.
  The 7 Habits of Highly Effective People
  Principle-Centered Leadership

Frankl, Victor
  Man's Search for Meaning

Hill, Napoleon
  Think and Grow Rich

Jampolsky, Gerald
  Love is Letting Go of Fear

Mandino, Og
  Mission Success
  The Greatest Salesman in the World
  The Greatest Success in the World

McGinnis, Alan Loy
  The Friendship Factor
  Bringing Out the Best in People

Peale, Norman Vincent
  The Power of Positive Thinking
  Bible Power for Successful Living

Robbins, Anthony
  Unlimited Power
  Awaken the Giant Within

Seligman, Martin
Learned Optimism
What You Can Change and What You Can't

Waitley, Denis
The Double Win
Being the Best
Seeds of Greatness

Ziglar, Zig
Confession of a Happy Christian
See You at the Top
Top Performance

CHAPTER THREE

KEY #3—POSITIVE RELATIONSHIPS

STEP 1.

Learn to help others

STEP 2.

Develop positive qualities

STEP 3.

Learn to listen

STEP 4.

Find the good

STEP 5.

Demonstrate love and appreciation

STEP 6.

Develop intimacy

STEP 7.

Recognize challenges in relationships

KEY #3—POSITIVE RELATIONSHIPS

Human beings need each other. We need to work with others, exchange services, share information, and provide emotional comfort. Positive human relationships sustain us and nourish us —body and soul.

Without positive human relationships, we cannot be healthy. What happens when we're cut off from others? In an experiment cited in *Bible Power for Successful Living,* by Norman Vincent Peale, a hospital staff assessed the impact of isolation on their own mascot. This dog had typically been lavished with attention and affection. When staff members made a small incision in a bone in the dog's leg, they found it in healthy, pink condition.

After the first incision, the hospital staff ignored the dog for a few days. They stopped petting it or paying it any attention. The dog was miserable. They made another small incision, and found that the interior of the bone was brown and dry.

Finally, the staff started to greet and pet the dog as they had done originally. When they made the third incision, once more the bone tissue looked pink and healthy.

This situation brings to mind Proverbs 17:22, "A merry heart doeth good like medicine: but a broken spirit drieth the bones."

Loneliness affects us—even on a cellular level. In fact, poor personal relationships and lack of social support can actually damage the immune system, according to *Mind/Body Medicine,* edited by Daniel Goleman, Ph.D., and Joel Gurin. Researchers who have studied diverse groups of people have found that those who are lonely—as assessed by psychological tests—are more likely to have sluggish immune systems.

There's still more evidence that loneliness can make us sick. Sociologist James House and colleagues investigated data from large, well-controlled population studies. They concluded that unsatisfactory social relationships were as important a risk factor for heart disease and premature death as smoking, high blood pressure, high blood cholesterol, obesity, and inactivity.

If loneliness leads to illness, it makes sense that love and positive human relationships are truly the road to health. In a study of almost 7,000 adults in Alameda County, California, researchers

Lisa Berkman, Ph.D., and S. Leonard Syme, Ph.D., found that people with more social contacts were two to five times more likely to outlive their more isolated counterparts.

At Tel Aviv University in Israel, a five-year study of almost 10,000 men diagnosed as having high risk of heart disease found they were almost twice as likely not to develop angina pectoris— chest pain from restriction of blood to the heart—if they felt they had loving and supportive wives. Researchers were surprised to discover that other risk factors, including hypertension and high cholesterol, were also significantly reduced if a husband believed he had his wife's love and support.

Dr. Ken Pelletier, of the University of California, San Francisco, School of Medicine, and author of *Mind as Healer, Mind as Slayer* says, "Community support groups and close personal relationships have been linked to better health and lower absenteeism, lower incidence of cancer and heart disease, and reduced hospital stays." In one study cited by Dr. Pelletier, researchers divided 1,337 medical students into two groups: one made up of students who were not close to their parents and were dissatisfied with their personal relationships, and one that was psychologically healthier. The first group was found to have a three to four times higher risk of cancer later in life than the healthier students.

Dr. Pelletier pointed out that people who feel they don't have enough social support are more susceptible to arthritis, tuberculosis, high blood pressure, and heart disease. He stated, "There is a link between disease and depression, loneliness, and hopelessness that's been shown in research."

A community that demonstrated the health benefits of the ties that bind was Roseto, Pennsylvania. A study published in the *American Journal of Public Health* showed that in this closely knit community of Italian-Americans, despite their high-fat diet, heart disease rates were significantly lower than those in neighboring towns and the rest of the United States. However, when younger members moved away from the community, their rate of heart disease climbed substantially and began to equal national norms.

This appears to be true all over the world. People in Japan are known for their strong attachment to community. They also enjoy the longest life expectancy in the world. And people in less developed societies who are close to their neighbors have lower blood pressure and fewer symptoms of heart problems than individuals in more advanced societies, who are more distant from their neighbors. Is this coincidence? I don't think so.

Do the negative feelings themselves cause illness, or are unhappy people less inclined to take good care of themselves? Perhaps the distinction is immaterial. If we can take control of our thoughts and feelings, perhaps we can learn to take greater control of our health.

Step 1. *Learn to help others*

Altruism is defined as unselfish concern for the welfare of others. Although its focus is on others, altruistic love does serve the self indirectly by promoting health.

Allan Luks, former executive director of the Institute for the Advancement of Health, distributed questionnaires to 3,000 volunteers. He found that "People who help others frequently report better health than people who don't." He also found that over 90% of respondents reported positive physical sensations linked to helping others: exhilaration, strength, and tranquility. Kathy Keeton, author of *Longevity*, writes, "It's becoming increasingly clear that a helpful, caring attitude toward others may be a ticket not only to a happier and more productive life, but to a longer life as well."

There's a universal truth that too few people in this world really believe in: By helping others, we help ourselves. In Chapter 1, Step 5, I urged you to begin as a servant of others. Adopting this attitude will produce dramatic changes in the quality of your life, especially in your personal relationships.

Here is a story from Zig Ziglar's *See You at the Top* that really demonstrates how important it is for us to help one another.

> "A man was given a tour of both Heaven and Hell, so he could intelligently select his final destination. The Devil was given first chance, so he started the 'prospect' with a tour of Hell. The first glance was a surprising one because all occupants were seated at a banquet table loaded with every food imaginable, including meat from every corner

of the globe, fruits and vegetables and every delicacy known to man. With justification, the Devil pointed out that no one could ask for more.

"However, when the man looked carefully at the people he did not find a single smile. He heard no music nor did he see any indication of the gaiety generally associated with such a feast. The people at the table looked dull and listless and were literally skin and bones. The tourist noticed that each person had a fork strapped to the left arm and a knife strapped to the right arm. Each had a four-foot handle which made it impossible to eat. So, with food of every kind at their fingertips, they were starving.

"Next stop was Heaven, where the tourist saw a scene identical in every respect—same foods, same knives and forks with those four-foot handles. However, the inhabitants of Heaven were laughing, singing, and having a great time. They were well fed and in excellent health. The tourist was puzzled for a moment. He wondered how conditions could be so similar and yet produce such different results. The people in Hell were starving and miserable, while the people in Heaven were well-fed and happy. Then, he saw the reason. Each person in Hell had been trying to feed himself. A knife and fork with a four-foot handle made this impossible. Each person in Heaven was feeding the one across the table from him and was being fed by the one sitting on the opposite side. By helping one another, they helped themselves."

The point of this story is clear. It highlights Zig Ziglar's message: *You can get everything in life you want, if you help enough people get what they want.* If you want more love in your life, give more love. If you want more acceptance in your life, become more accepting of others. Whatever you want, you have to give it first before you can receive.

STEP 2. *Develop positive qualities*

What traits do you value in other people? What are the positive qualities of a friend? A very special friend of mine sent me a fax one day. He had come across a poem and wrote that it made him think of me. After reading the poem, I felt truly honored.

A Friend...
Someone with whom you can share your inner feelings...
    knowing you won't be judged or rejected.
Someone who gives freely...
    without expectation or motivation.
Someone who lets you be who you are...
    if you want to change, it's up to you.
Someone who is there when you're hurting...
    offering true tenderness.
Someone who sees your beauty...
    your true beauty.
Someone who gives you space when it's
    needed...without hesitation.
Someone who listens...
    to what you are really saying.
Someone who will consider your different
    beliefs...without judgment.
Someone whom you always feel close to...
    even when they are far away.
Someone with whom you feel comfortable...
    anytime, anywhere, doing anything.
A friend is a special gift...
    to be cherished forever.

        —Datus

We all need the love and acceptance of friends and family. In order to meet these needs, we must first develop the positive qualities of friendship within ourselves. In other words, in order to have a friend, we must first be a friend. Many of the qualities needed are stated in the poem above. Let me list some of the positive qualities I admire in people and strive to attain:

- Honesty
- Integrity
- Humility
- Dependability

- Loyalty
- Sincerity
- Enthusiasm
- Hard-working

- Open-mindedness
- A sense of humor
- Dedication

The great news is that these positive qualities can be learned or developed. Develop the characteristics of a true friend deep within you, and you will be blessed with very gratifying and rewarding relationships—ones that will nourish your body, mind, and soul.

STEP 3. *Learn to listen*

The quality of any relationship ultimately comes down to the quality of its communication. The biggest roadblock to effective communication in most relationships is poor listening skills. I really believe that "listening is loving." When we are truly listening, we are telling the person that he or she is important to us and that we respect and love him or her. Here are seven tips to good listening that I found easy to learn and quite useful.

Tip #1

Do not interrupt. Allow the person you are communicating with to really share his feelings and thoughts uninterrupted. Empathize with him, put yourself in his shoes. If you first seek to understand, you will find yourself being better understood.

Tip #2

Be an active listener. This means that you must act really interested in what the other person is communicating. Listen to what she is saying instead of thinking about your response. Ask questions to gain more information or clarify what she is telling you. Good questions open lines of communication.

Tip #3

Be a reflective listener. Restate or reflect back to the other person your interpretation of what he is telling you. This simple technique shows the other person that you are both listening and understanding what he is saying. Restating what you think is being said may cause some short-term conflict in some situations, but is certainly worth the risk. Just explain that you want to be certain you understand what he is trying to say.

Tip #4

Wait to speak until the person or people you want to communicate with are listening. If they are not ready to listen, no matter how well you communicate, your message will not be heard.

Tip #5

Don't try to talk over somebody. If you find yourself being interrupted, relax. Don't try to out-talk the other person. If you are courteous and allow him to speak, eventually (unless he is extremely rude), he will respond likewise. If he doesn't, point out to him that he is interrupting the communication process. You can only do this if you have been a good listener. Double standards in relationships seldom work.

Tip #6

Help the other person become an active listener. This can be done by asking her if she understood what you were communicating. Ask her to tell you what she heard. If she doesn't seem to be understanding what you are saying, keep after it until she does.

Tip #7

Don't be afraid of long silences. Human communication involves much more than words. Unfortunately, in many situations silence can make us feel uncomfortable, but a great deal can be communicated during silences. Relax. Some people need silence to collect their thoughts and feel safe in communicating. The important thing to remember during silences is that you must remain an active listener.

STEP 4. *Find the good*

The way you see others has an effect on how you relate to them, how they view you, and how you view yourself. I urge you to become what Zig Ziglar calls a "good finder"—someone who looks for the good in other people or situations. In *See You at the Top,* Zig tells the story of an experiment conducted at Harvard University by Dr. Robert Rosenthal. A series of tests involving three groups of students and three groups of rats were conducted under the supervision of Dr. Rosenthal. He informed the first group of students, "You're in luck. You are going to be working with genius rats. These rats have been bred for intelligence and are extremely bright. They will run through the maze with great ease."

The second group was told, "Your rats are just average. They are not too bright, not too dumb, just a bunch of average rats. Don't expect too much from them, because they are just average."

The third group was told, "Your rats are really dumb. If they find the end of the maze, it will be purely by accident."

For the next six weeks, the students timed the performance of individual rats running through the maze. Not surprisingly, the genius rats behaved like geniuses and had the lowest times. The average rats were average and the dumb rats were really dumb.

What is so amazing about this study? Well, it turns out that all of the rats were from the same litter. There were no genius, average, or dumb rats. The only difference between them was the direct result of the difference in attitude and expectations of the students conducting the experiments.

Does the same thing happen with humans? Most definitely. Studies conducted with teachers and children produced the same kind of results as the studies with the rats. Remarkable as it may seem, it has been shown many times in controlled experiments that parents, teachers, managers, and others will get exactly what they expect. This phenomenon is called the "Pygmalion Effect."

According to Greek mythology, Pygmalion was a sculptor and King of Cyprus who fell in love with one of his creations. The ivory statue came to life after Pygmalion's repeated prayers to the Goddess of Love, Venus. Pygmalion's vision was so powerful and his faith so strong, his vision became his reality. The myth exemplifies the truth that what we see reflected in many objects, situations, or persons is what we put there with our own expectations. We create images of how things should be, and if these images are believed, they become self-fulfilling prophecies.

If we expect only the worst from people, that is exactly what we see. If we focus our attention on the positives, if we look for the good in people and situations, that becomes our reality. In addition, if we are constantly criticizing and looking for the negatives in people, this attitude is reflected. We too are harshly judged, criticized, and not very well liked.

To be happy and have positive relationships, you absolutely must become a good finder. You must look for the good in people. You must expect the best from people. And, you must reinforce the good that you see. You must demonstrate your love and appreciation.

STEP 5. *Demonstrate love and appreciation*

It is not enough to simply feel love in our friendships and intimate relationships. We must express these feelings. We must demonstrate to our loved ones just how important they are to us. We must continually find ways to communicate our deepest feelings through our actions, whether they be verbal, written, through touch, or by our behavior. We all need to see, hear, and physically feel loved and appreciated.

What are some ways to express love and appreciation? The most direct is to tell the person face-to-face or with a card or letter. Think of some times in your life when you felt really loved or appreciated. What made you feel that way? If a certain action produced a feeling of being loved and appreciated within you, it is likely that a similar action will produce those same feelings in another person. What a phenomenal gift you can give! I strongly urge you to seek out ways to continually tell those around you how much you love and appreciate them. Again, it is important to remember that what we give out, we get back.

STEP 6. *Develop intimacy*

Intimacy is very important to good health. It probably relates to the nurturing that takes place when we share our deepest selves. Intimate relationships are the most gratifying. However, many people have a hard time developing a truly intimate relationship—especially with their spouse. Friendships can be intimate, but our most intimate relationship is usually with our spouse or "significant other." The benefit here is that in addition to emotional intimacy, we also share physical intimacy.

Here are three simple tips to help nourish intimacy between friends or lovers:

Tip #1

Take a walk together. Moving together physically really opens up communication. It has to do with body language and a phenomenon called "mirroring and matching." Adopting another person's speech, body language, or behavior triggers our subconscious to develop a feeling of rapport. The next time you are out in a restaurant, take a look around and notice how many people (especially lovers) are mirroring and matching. You'll be amazed. Try using mirroring and matching to your advantage to enhance intimacy. It is very powerful.

Tip #2

Ask questions which open communication and let your partner answer the questions fully. This tip is extremely useful when challenges present themselves. The key is to frame questions in a positive light and allow your partner to really express him or herself. For example, when you ask your partner what kind of a day he or she had, listen to the feelings behind the words. Try to hear any concerns he or she might want to talk out. When something good happens, let your partner know how delighted you are for his success, how proud you are of her accomplishment. Let him or her expound. Really listen!

Tip #3

Find an activity that you both enjoy and do it together. Whether it is going to a movie, playing a game, eating at a favorite restaurant, or taking a drive or a walk together, it doesn't matter, as long as it is something you both enjoy doing, and you are doing it together.

If you have few intimate relationships in your life, you need to reach out and establish more friendships. Here are four additional tips you may find useful:

Tip #4

Look for opportunities to extend the contacts you make through your church, fitness center, or community program.

Tip #5

Attend workshops, seminars, and classes you are interested in. You will find people who share your beliefs and interests—fertile ground for developing supportive friendships.

Tip #6

Become a volunteer at your local hospital, school, nursing home, or any other place where you can really make a difference.

Tip #7

Get a pet. A relationship with a pet can be almost as positive as a human relationship. Studies have shown that owning or caring for a pet can relieve loneliness, depression, and anxiety, and even promote a quicker recovery from illness.

STEP 7. *Recognize challenges in relationships*

Any good relationship is going to be faced with challenges. It is from these challenges that the relationship will either be enhanced, nourished, and encouraged to grow—or be destroyed. A relationship based on love, trust, honesty, respect, and other positive values will survive any challenge; however, a relationship that lacks a strong foundation may crumble after even a very minor challenge.

Most challenges in relationships are the result of incomplete or misunderstood communications. In her book, *Making Love All of the Time*, Dr. Barbara De Angelis identifies four phases that can kill a relationship. By recognizing these four phases, you can prevent challenges from escalating to a level which can destroy the relationship. Here are the four phases:

Stage One—Resistance

The first phase of a relationship challenge is resistance. Resistance occurs when you take exception or feel annoyed or a bit separate from this person. It's nothing major, but if not effectively dealt with by loving communication, resistance can turn into resentment.

Stage Two—Resentment

The seed of resistance has flowered into a stronger negative feeling—resentment. You are not just annoyed; feelings of anger are present and an emotional barrier develops that destroys intimacy. If not dealt with, resentment then turns into rejection.

Stage Three—Rejection

In this phase, everything your partner does irritates or annoys you. Little meaningless things grow into huge conflicts. Rejection means emotional separation, yet it is quite painful. If not dealt with, rejection then turns into repression.

Stage Four—Repression

When you are tired of coping with the anger that comes with the rejection phase, repressing emotions becomes a mechanism to deal with the pain. Although pain is somewhat avoided, so is love, passion, and excitement. Couples become more like roommates than lovers in this phase.

Recognizing these four phases is the first step in preventing them from destroying a relationship. When you find yourself in one of these phases, it is critical to eliminate the negative feelings by addressing their source. Trying to sweep things under a rug or ignoring them only makes things worse.

The key to avoiding or getting out of this spiral of negative feelings is communication. Explain clearly the specific instance that is bothering you, but remember to ask questions in a positive light and really listen to your partner. Chances are both of you are feeling cut off, hurt, rejected. Try to empathize with the hurt inside your partner. When you listen with love and concern, doors open.

A relationship takes commitment from both parties. You must both be committed to learning how to communicate and behave in a manner consistent with your feelings. This small price is well worth the bounty of rewards that comes from positive relationships.

CHAPTER FOUR

KEY #4—A HEALTHY LIFESTYLE

STEP 1.

Do not smoke

STEP 2.

Do not drink or drink only in moderation

STEP 3.

Get adequate rest

STEP 4.

Learn to deal with stress effectively

STEP 5.

Learn to manage time effectively

STEP 6.

Connect with nature

STEP 7.

Laugh long and often

KEY #4—A HEALTHY LIFESTYLE

The United States Surgeon General's publication, *Health Promotion and Disease Prevention*, reported on an analysis of the ten leading causes of death in the U.S. It clearly showed that the majority of all early deaths are related to diet and lifestyle. This chapter focuses on the necessary steps involved in creating a healthy lifestyle.

A healthy lifestyle improves the quality and longevity of life. Currently, the life expectancy for men is 71 years, and for women, it is 78 years. Increasing life expectancy involves reducing the causes of premature death. The major killers are now heart disease, cancer and strokes. As more people make the necessary dietary and lifestyle changes to reduce their risk of these diseases, life expectancy in the United States should continue to increase.

STEP 1. *Do not smoke*

Cigarette smoking is one of the major factors contributing to premature death in the United States. Health experts have determined that cigarette smoking is the single major cause of cancer death in the United States. Cigarette smokers have total, overall cancer death rates twice that of non-smokers. The greater the number of cigarettes smoked, the greater the risk.

Smoking also increases the risk of death from heart attacks and strokes. In fact, according to the U.S. Surgeon General, "Cigarette smoking should be considered the most important risk factor for coronary heart disease." Statistical evidence reveals a three-to-fivefold increase in the risk of coronary artery disease in smokers compared to non-smokers. The more cigarettes smoked and the longer a person has smoked, the greater the risk of dying from a heart attack or stroke. Overall, the average smoker dies seven to eight years sooner than the non-smoker.

If you want good health, you absolutely must stop smoking! Here are eleven tips to help you stop:

Tip #1
List all the reasons why you want to quit smoking
and review them daily.

Tip #2

Set a specific day to quit, tell at least ten friends that you are going to quit smoking, and then DO IT!

Tip #3

Throw away all cigarettes, butts, matches, and ashtrays.

Tip #4

Use substitutes. Instead of smoking, chew on raw vegetables, fruits, or gum. If your fingers seem empty, play with a pencil.

Tip #5

Take one day at a time.

Tip #6

Realize that more than 40 million Americans have quit. If they can do it, so can you!

Tip #7

Visualize yourself as a non-smoker with a fatter pocketbook, pleasant breath, unstained teeth, and the satisfaction that comes from being in control of your life.

Tip #8

Join a support group. Call the local American Cancer Society and ask for referrals. You are not alone.

Tip #9

When you need to relax, perform deep breathing exercises rather than reaching for a cigarette.

Tip #10

Avoid situations that you associate with smoking.

Tip #11

Each day, reward yourself in a positive way. Buy yourself something with the money you've saved or plan a special reward as a celebration for quitting.

STEP 2. *Do not drink or drink only in moderation*

Alcohol is our nation's number one drug problem as it seriously affects the health of more than 10 million people. While moderate drinking (no more than one or two drinks per day) has actually been shown to be associated with a longer life, excessive drinking is strongly associated with five of the leading causes of death in the United States: accidents, cirrhosis of the liver, pneumonia, suicide, and murder.

Consequences of alcohol abuse

Increased mortality:
- 10-year decrease in life expectancy
- Double the usual death rate in men, triple in women
- Six times greater suicide rate
- Major contributing factor in the four leading causes of death in men between the ages of 25 and 44: accidents, homicides, suicides, cirrhosis

Economic toll (yearly):
- Lost production: over $20 billion
- Health care costs: over $10 billion
- Accident and fire losses: $5 billion
- Cost of violent crime: $4 billion

Health effects:
- Metabolic damage to every cell
- Intoxication
- Abstinence and withdrawal syndromes
- Nutritional diseases
- Brain damage
- Psychiatric disorders
- Esophagitis, gastritis, ulcer
- Increased cancer of mouth, pharynx, larynx, esophagus
- Pancreatitis
- Liver fatty degeneration and cirrhosis
- Heart disease
- High blood pressure

- Angina
- Hypoglycemia
- Decreased protein synthesis
- Increased serum and liver triglycerides
- Decreased serum testosterone
- Muscle damage
- Osteoporosis
- Birth defects

If you think you have a drinking problem, seek out help. Contact your local Alcoholics Anonymous or similar program. Also, I have found that many alcoholics have faulty control over blood sugar levels. People who crave sugar and alcohol can benefit by eating small, frequent meals and taking a formula like Enzymatic Therapy's Hypo-Ade, which provides essential nutrients required by the body to regulate blood sugar levels.

STEP 3. *Get adequate rest*

Are you getting enough sleep? If not, your health may be suffering. Sufficient sleep and rest are essential to good health. Your body needs sleep to function properly. During sleep, the body repairs itself. Without sufficient sleep, needed repairs go undone, and the body is more likely to break down.

During sleep, your body systems undergo major positive changes. For example:

- brain waves slow down
- blood pressure falls
- muscles relax
- the pituitary gland produces more hormones
- immune function is enhanced
- your body actively repairs damaged tissues and cells
- you dream, allowing your mind to work out unresolved psychological and emotional issues

Exactly how much sleep you need depends upon you. Some people find they need only 5 or 6 hours of sleep; others may need 10 or 11. Regardless of how much sleep you think you might require, the truth is most Americans do not get enough sleep to function optimally. In addition, at least 40 million Americans suffer from insomnia or some other sleep disturbance.

To improve your ability to sleep, give yourself some time to wind down before going to bed. Avoid stimulants such as caffeine or television programs that keep you on the edge of your seat. Sip some herbal tea and listen to some beautiful music or a relaxation tape. Let the day go. Whatever you must accomplish tomorrow, give yourself permission to rest now, so you'll wake with the energy needed to get the job done.

STEP 4. *Learn to deal with stress effectively*

Stress is common in our fast-paced society. Often the demands placed on us daily build until it is almost impossible to cope. Job pressures. Family arguments. Financial pressures. Deadlines. These are common examples of "stressors." Actually, a stressor can be anything that creates a disturbance within our body: exposure to heat or cold, environmental toxins, toxins produced by micro-organisms, physical trauma, and, of course, strong emotions.

Some basic control mechanisms are geared toward counter-acting the everyday stresses of life. The initial response to stress is the alarm reaction, or "flight or fight" response. Triggered by reactions in the brain which cause the adrenal glands to secrete adrenaline and other stress-related hormones, the fight or flight response is designed to counteract danger by mobilizing the body's resources for immediate physical activity. This is great if you need to escape from a tiger or some other life-threatening situation. However, if stress is extreme, unusual, or long-lasting, the effects of these mechanisms can be quite harmful.

Conditions strongly linked to psychological stress
- Angina
- Asthma
- Autoimmune disease
- Cancer
- Cardiovascular disease
- Common cold
- Depression
- Diabetes
- Headaches (adult onset, Type II)

- Hypertension
- Immune system suppression
- Irritable bowel
- Menstrual syndrome irregularities
- Premenstrual tension
- Rheumatoid arthritis syndrome
- Ulcerative colitis
- Ulcers

Specific relaxation techniques can reduce the amount of stress. (For example, I have described a relaxation/visualization exercise on pages 30 and 31.) More important than the type of relaxation technique is that you set aside at least 10 to 15 minutes each day to do it.

Although you can relax by simply sleeping, watching television, or reading a book, relaxation techniques are designed specifically to produce the physiological state Herbert Benson, M.D., describes in his best-selling book, *The Relaxation Response.* The physiological effects of the relaxation response are opposite to those seen with stress.

In the stress response, the sympathetic nervous system dominates. In the relaxation response, the parasympathetic nervous system dominates. The parasympathetic nervous system controls body functions such as digestion, breathing, and heart rate during periods of rest, relaxation, visualization, meditation, and sleep. While the sympathetic nervous system is designed to protect us against immediate danger, the parasympathetic system is designed for repair, maintenance, and restoration of the body.

Producing deep relaxation with any relaxation technique requires learning how to breathe. Have you ever noticed how a baby breathes? With each breath, the baby's abdomen rises and falls because the baby is breathing with its diaphragm, a dome-shaped muscle that separates the chest cavity from the abdominal cavity. If you are like most adults, you tend to fill only your upper chest because you do not utilize the diaphragm. Shallow breathing tends to produce tension and fatigue.

One of the most powerful methods of producing less stress and more energy in the body is breathing with the diaphragm. By using the diaphragm to breathe, you can dramatically change your physiology. Diaphragmatic breathing literally activates the relaxation centers in the brain. Here is a popular technique I use to train people to breathe using their diaphragm.

- Find a quiet, comfortable place to lie down or sit.
- Place your feet slightly apart. Place one hand on your abdomen near your navel. Place the other hand on your chest.
- You will be inhaling through your nose and exhaling through your mouth.
- Concentrate on your breathing. Note which hand is rising and falling with each breath.
- Gently exhale most of the air in your lungs.
- Inhale while slowly counting to 4. As you inhale, slightly extend your abdomen, causing it to rise about one inch. Make sure that you are not moving your chest or shoulders.
- As you inhale, imagine the warmed air flowing in. Imagine its warmth flowing to all parts of your body.
- Pause for one second, then slowly exhale to a count of 4. As you exhale, your abdomen should move inward.
- As the air flows out, imagine all the tension and stress leaving your body.
- Repeat the process until a sense of deep relaxation is achieved.

Now that you know how to breathe, the important thing is to remember to breathe with your diaphragm as much as possible—especially during times of increased stress—and to perform a relaxation technique for 10 to 15 minutes each day.

STEP 5. *Learn to manage time effectively*

One of the biggest stressors for most people is time. They simply do not feel they have enough of it. Here are some tips on time management that really seem to work. Oh, by the way, time management does not mean squeezing more and more work into less and less time. It means learning to plan your time more effectively, so you can do the activities in life that you enjoy.

Tip #1

Set priorities. Realize that you can only accomplish so much in a day. Decide what is important, and limit your efforts to that goal.

Tip #2

Organize your day. Interruptions and unplanned demands on your time will always occur, but create a definite plan for the day based on your priorities. Avoid the pitfall of allowing the "immediate demands" to control your life.

Tip #3

Delegate authority. Delegate as much authority and work as you can. You can't do everything yourself. Learn to train and depend on others.

Tip #4

Tackle the toughest job first. Handle the most important tasks first while your energy levels are high. Leave the busywork or running around for later in the day.

Tip #5

Minimize meeting time. Schedule meetings to bump up against the lunch hour or quitting time; that way they can't last forever.

Tip #6

Avoid putting things off. Work done under pressure of an unreasonable deadline often has to be redone. That creates more stress than if it had been done right the first time. Plan ahead.

Tip #7

Don't be a perfectionist. You can never really achieve perfection anyway. Do your best in a reasonable amount of time, then move on to other important tasks. If you find time, you can always come back later and polish the task some more.

Step 6. *Connect with nature*

Most Americans spend 90% of their lives indoors separated from fresh air, natural sunlight, and nature. Something extremely refreshing and calming happens when we can get in touch with nature, whether it is simply a walk through a park or getting out in the wilderness for a weekend of camping. Personally, I find the rhythms and sounds of nature very relaxing. Since I can't always get out and enjoy nature as much as I would like, I do the next best thing—I listen to sounds of nature.

In my office, car, and home, I usually have a recording of sounds of nature playing in the background. The recordings are of beautifully relaxing music intertwined with sounds of nature, like the sounds at an isolated beach, waterfall, or forest. I find myself being more productive and relaxed when these gentle sounds are playing. I highly recommend it.

Step 7. *Laugh long and often*

The late Norman Cousins' popular book *Anatomy of an Illness* caused a significant stir in the medical community in 1979. Cousins' book provided an autobiographical anecdotal account of how laughter and positive emotional states can help heal the body, even of quite serious disease. Cousins watched *Candid Camera* and Marx brothers films, and read humorous books.

Originally physicians and researchers scoffed at Cousins' account. Now, however, numerous studies have demonstrated that laughter and other positive emotional states can, in fact, enhance the immune system. Recent medical research has also confirmed that laughter:

- enhances blood flow to the body's extremities and improves cardiovascular function,
- plays an active part in the body's release of endorphins and other natural mood-elevating and pain-killing chemicals, and
- improves the transfer of oxygen and nutrients to internal organs.

By laughing frequently and taking a lighter view of life, you will find that life is much more enjoyable and fun. Here are eight tips to help you get more laughter in your life.

Tip #1
Learn to laugh at yourself.

Recognize how funny some of your behavior really is—especially your shortcomings or mistakes. I am really lucky because I have many little foibles and goofs that make me laugh at myself. And, I work at Enzymatic Therapy, a great place where people accept me for who I am, but can point out little things I do that are funny.

For example, I have trouble saying certain words. When I say specific, it comes out "pecific." I don't know why or how it comes out this way, but it almost always does. Most people wouldn't even notice, but at staff meetings when I am talking about our Liquid Liver Extract which is derived from a "specific" fraction of bovine liver— it seems everyone notices and gets a good laugh in, including myself. Hey, we are all human. We all have little idiosyncrasies or behaviors that are unique to us that we can recognize and enjoy.

I must point out that there is a big difference between laughing *with* others and laughing *at* others. Because of the atmosphere at Enzymatic Therapy and the values of the company and its employees, I know that when I say "pecific," people are not laughing at me, they are laughing with me. I am included in the laughter because I can laugh at myself. In fact, now that I am aware of it, I will often exaggerate and say that our Liquid Liver Extract is from a "pecific" fraction of bovine liver just to lighten up the mood of a meeting.

Tip #2
Inject humor anytime it is appropriate.

I just gave an example of injecting humor into a meeting. At Enzymatic Therapy, humor abounds. Consultants who come into our offices are amazed at how productive our staff is and how much they seem to be enjoying their work. They are amazed to sit in on our executive meetings and observe us laughing regularly, yet still accomplishing our meeting goals. I explain to them that I believe we are accomplishing our goals and objectives so well because of our enjoyment of each other and the whole process.

Humor and laughter really make work enjoyable. We have employees who cannot wait to get to work because they have so much fun in their jobs. I want my employees to be happy. I believe they have to be free to inject humor into their work in order to be happy. They have the freedom to socialize and share among themselves as long as they get their work done. While some managers might look at such behavior as "goofing off," I recognize the importance of humor in developing good morale and greater productivity.

Tip #3
Read the comics to find one that
you like and follow it.

Humor is very individual. What I may find funny, you may not, but the comics or "funny papers" have something for everybody. Read them thoroughly to find a comic strip that strikes you as particularly funny and look for it every day or week.

Tip #4
Watch comedies on television.

With modern cable systems, I am amazed at how easy it is to find something funny on television. When I am in need of a good laugh, I try to find something I can laugh at on TV. Some of my favorites are the old-time classics like *Andy Griffith, Gilligan's Island, Mary Tyler Moore*, etc. If I can't find anything on TV, then I will watch something from my VCR collection. I have collected all of the *Andy Griffith* shows because no matter how many times I see an episode, it always makes me laugh or feel good inside.

Tip #5

Go to comedies at the movie theater.

I love to go to the movies, especially a comedy. It is not just my personal enjoyment of the movie that I like. What I enjoy most is going to the movie with my family or friends because their companionship really enhances the whole experience. If we see a funny movie together, I find myself laughing harder and longer. We feed off each other's laughter during and after the movie. Sharing a funny movie together means that we will be talking about specific (there is that word again) scenes from the movie that really made us laugh.

Tip #6

Listen to comedy audiotapes in your car while commuting.

Check your local record or book store, video store, or library for recorded comedy routines of your favorite comic. If you haven't heard or seen many comics, go to your library first. You'll find an abundance of tapes to investigate, and you can check them out for free.

Tip #7

Play with kids.

Kids really know how to laugh and play. If you do not have kids of your own, spend time with your nieces, nephews, or neighborhood children with whose families you are friendly. Become a Big Brother or Big Sister. Investigate local Little Leagues. Help out at your church's Sunday School and children's events.

Tip #8

Ask yourself, "What is funny about this situation?"

Many times we will find ourselves in seemingly impossible situations, but, if we can laugh about them, somehow they become enjoyable or at least tolerable experiences. One time, Dr. Murray and I were visiting some companies in Europe, and we found ourselves in an interesting situation. We had gotten on an express train going in the opposite direction of where we were supposed to be headed. Express trains are so-called because they only make stops at large cities many miles apart.

Our immediate reaction was to break out into almost uncontrollable laughter. We immediately recognized the humor of our situation and realized we were powerless to stop the train and turn it around. We could only accept our mistake, wait for the next stop (about an hour), and board a new train going in the right direction.

Some people would have become angry or started asking negative questions like, "How could we be so stupid?" or "What did we do to deserve this?" Or, they would have tried to delegate blame (by the way, it was Dr. Murray's fault—just kidding, Mike). Instead of a "negative" experience, Dr. Murray and I were given another experience that we can reflect back on with a good laugh.

So many times, I have heard people say, "This is something you will look back on and laugh about." Well, why wait—find the humor in the situation and enjoy a good laugh immediately.

Chapter Five

Key #5—Regular Exercise

Step 1.
Realize the importance of physical exercise

Step 2.
Consult your physician

Step 3.
Select an activity you can enjoy

Step 4.
Monitor your exercise intensity

Step 5.
Do it often

Step 6.
Make it fun

Step 7.
Stay motivated

KEY #5—REGULAR EXERCISE

Regular physical exercise is obviously a vital key to good health. We all know this fact, yet only a small fraction (less than 20%) of Americans exercise on a regular basis. Why? Excuses like lack of time, lack of energy, or lack of motivation are frequently given. Are these excuses valid? How important is your health? How important is regular exercise to your overall health?

Exercise is absolutely vital. While the immediate effect of exercise is stress on the body, with regular exercise the body adapts—it becomes stronger, functions more efficiently, and has greater endurance. The entire body benefits from regular exercise, largely as a result of improved cardiovascular and respiratory functions. Simply stated, exercise enhances the transport of oxygen and nutrients into cells. At the same time, exercise enhances the transport of carbon dioxide and waste products from the tissues of the body to the bloodstream and ultimately to the eliminative organs. As a result, regular exercise increases stamina and energy levels.

Regular exercise is particularly important in reducing the risk of heart disease. It does this by lowering cholesterol levels, improving blood and oxygen supply to the heart, increasing the functional capacity of the heart, reducing blood pressure, reducing obesity, and exerting a favorable effect on blood clotting.

Physical inactivity is a major reason why so many Americans are overweight. This is especially true in children. Studies have demonstrated that childhood obesity is associated more with inactivity than overeating. Since strong evidence suggests that 80 to 86% of adult obesity begins in childhood, it can be concluded that lack of physical activity is a major cause of obesity.

People who are physically active tend to have less of a problem with weight loss. Regular exercise is a necessary component of any effective weight-loss program due to the following factors:

1. When weight loss is achieved by dieting without exercise, a substantial portion of the total weight loss comes from the lean tissue, primarily as water loss.

2. When exercise is included in a weight-loss program, body composition improves. Lean body weight increases because of an increase in muscle mass and a decrease in body fat. Since muscle burns calories while fat is inert, an increase in muscle mass means your body is burning more calories all day long—even while you're asleep.

3. Exercise helps counter the reduction in basal metabolic rate (BMR)—the rate at which your body burns calories when you're inactive or at rest—that usually accompanies dieting alone and, in Western society, aging.

4. Exercise increases the BMR not just when you're exercising, but for an extended period of time following the exercise session.

5. Moderate to intense exercise may help suppress the appetite.

6. People who exercise during and after weight reduction are better able to maintain their weight loss than those who do not exercise.

Exercise is an efficient way to burn fat. Muscle tissue is the primary user of fat calories in the body, so the greater your muscle mass, the greater your fat-burning capacity. If you want to be healthy and achieve your ideal body weight, you must exercise.

Regular exercise also exerts a powerful positive effect on the mind. Tensions, depressions, feelings of inadequacy, and worries diminish greatly with regular exercise. Exercise alone has been demonstrated to have a tremendous impact on improving mood and the ability to handle life's stressful situations.

A study published in the *American Journal of Epidemiology* found that increased participation in exercise, sports, and physical activities is strongly associated with decreased symptoms of anxiety (restlessness, tension, etc.), depression (feelings that life is not worthwhile, low spirits, etc.), and malaise (rundown feeling, insomnia, etc.). Simply stated, people who participate in regular exercise have higher self-esteem, feel better, and are happier.

Regular exercise has been shown to enhance powerful mood-elevating substances in the brain known as endorphins. These compounds exert effects similar to morphine. In fact, their name (endo = endogenous, -rphins = morphines) was given to them because of their morphine-like effects. A clear association exists between exercise and endorphin elevation: When endorphins go up, mood follows.

Dennis Lobstein, Ph.D., a professor of exercise psychobiology at the University of New Mexico, compared the beta-endorphin levels and depression profiles of ten joggers versus ten sedentary men of the same age. The ten sedentary men tested out as more depressed, perceived greater stress in their lives, had more stress-circulating hormones and showed lower levels of beta-endorphins. As Dr. Lobstein stated, this "reaffirms that depression is very sensitive to exercise and helps firm up a biochemical link between physical activity and depression."

If the benefits of exercise could be put in a pill, you would have the most powerful health-promoting medication available. Take a look at this long list of health benefits produced by regular exercise:

Musculoskeletal system
- Increases muscle strength
- Increases flexibility of muscles and range of joint motion
- Produces stronger bones, ligaments, and tendons
- Lessens chance of injury
- Enhances posture, poise, and physique

Heart and blood vessels
- Lowers resting heart rate
- Strengthens heart function
- Lowers blood pressure
- Improves oxygen delivery throughout the body
- Increases blood supply to muscles
- Enlarges the arteries to the heart

Bodily processes
- Reduces heart disease risk
- Helps lower blood cholesterol and triglycerides
- Raises HDL, the "good" cholesterol

- Helps improve calcium deposition in bones
- Prevents osteoporosis
- Improves immune function
- Aids digestion and elimination
- Increases lean body mass
- Improves the body's ability to burn dietary fat
- Increases endurance and energy levels
- Increases strength
- Improves sensitivity to insulin
- Reduces risk of diabetes

Mental processes
- Provides a natural release for pent-up feelings
- Helps reduce tension and anxiety
- Improves mental outlook and self-esteem
- Helps relieve moderate depression
- Improves the ability to handle stress
- Stimulates improved mental function
- Relaxes and improves sleep
- Increases self-esteem

Longevity
- Research shows that for every hour of exercise we gain a two-hour increase in longevity

STEP 1. *Realize the importance of physical exercise*

The first step is realizing just how vital it is to your health to get regular exercise. But, even if you acknowledge this truth, unless you act on it by making regular exercise a top priority in your life, it means nothing.

STEP 2. *Consult your physician*

If you are not currently on a regular exercise program, get medical clearance if you have health problems or if you are over 40 years of age. The main concern is the functioning of your heart. Exercise can be quite harmful (even fatal) if your heart is not able to meet the increased demands placed upon it.

It is especially important to see a physician if any of the following applies to you:

- Heart disease
- Smoking
- High blood pressure
- Extreme breathlessness with physical exertion
- Pain or pressure in chest, arm, teeth, jaw or neck with exercise
- Dizziness or fainting
- Abnormal heart action (palpitations or irregular heartbeat)

STEP 3. *Select an activity you can enjoy*

If you are fit enough to begin, the next thing to do is select an activity that you feel you would enjoy. The best exercises are the kind that get your heart moving. Aerobic activities such as walking briskly, jogging, bicycling, cross-country skiing, swimming, aerobic dance, and racquet sports are good examples. Brisk walking (5 miles an hour) for approximately 30 minutes may be the very best form of exercise for most people. Walking can be done anywhere; it doesn't require any expensive equipment, just comfortable clothing and well-fitting shoes; and the risk of injury is extremely low. If you are going to walk on a regular basis, I strongly urge you to first purchase a pair of high-quality walking or jogging shoes. You'll be more comfortable, so you'll enjoy yourself more and will soon find you're walking longer and more frequently.

STEP 4. *Monitor your exercise intensity*

Exercise intensity is determined by measuring your heart rate (the number of times your heart beats per minute). This can be quickly determined by placing the index and middle finger of one hand on the side of your neck just below the angle of the jaw or on the opposite wrist. Beginning with zero, count the number of heartbeats for 6 seconds. Simply add a zero to this number and you have your pulse. For example, if you counted 14 beats, your heart rate would be 140. Would this be a good number? It depends upon your "training zone."

A quick and easy way to determine your maximum training heart rate is to simply subtract your age from 185. For example, if you are 40 years old, your maximum heart rate would be 145. To determine the bottom of the training zone, simply subtract 20 from this number. In the case of a 40-year-old, this would be 125. So, the training range would be between 125 and 145 beats per minute. For maximum health benefits, you must stay in this range and never exceed it.

STEP 5. *Do it often*

You don't get in good physical condition by exercising once. Exercise must be performed on a regular basis. A minimum of 15 to 20 minutes of exercising at your training heart rate at least three times a week is necessary to gain any significant cardiovascular benefits. Exercising at the lower end of your training zone for longer periods of time is much better than exercising at a higher intensity for a shorter period of time. It is also best if you can make exercise a part of your daily routine.

STEP 6. *Make it fun*

The key to getting the maximum benefit from exercise is to make it enjoyable. Choose an activity that you enjoy and have fun. If you can find enjoyment in exercise, you are much more likely to do it regularly. One way to make it fun is to get a workout partner. For example, if you choose walking as your activity, find one or two people at work or in your neighborhood with whom you would enjoy walking. If you are meeting someone else, you will certainly walk more regularly than if no one is depending on you. Commit to walking three to five mornings or afternoons each week, and increase the exercise duration from an initial 10 minutes to at least 30 minutes.

STEP 7. *Stay motivated*

No matter how committed a person is to regular exercise, at some point, he or she will lose enthusiasm for working out. Here is my suggestion—take a break. Not a long break, just skip one or two workouts. Give your enthusiasm and motivation a chance to recoup, so you can come back with an even stronger commitment.

Here are some things I do to keep myself motivated:

- Read or thumb through fitness magazines like *Men's Fitness*, *Muscle & Fitness*, and *Muscular Development*. Looking at pictures of people in fantastic shape really inspires me. In addition, these magazines typically feature articles on interesting new exercise routines I can try.

- Set exercise goals. Since I'm a goal-oriented individual, goals really help keep me motivated. Success breeds success, so make a lot of small goals that can easily be achieved. Write down your daily exercise goal and check it off when you have completed it.

- Vary your routine. Variety is important to keep exercise interesting. Doing the same thing every day becomes monotonous and drains motivation. Continually find new ways to enjoy working out.

- Keep a record of your activities and progress. Sometimes it is hard to see the progress you are making, but if you write in a journal, you'll have a permanent record of your progress. Seeing your progress in black and white will motivate you to continued improvement.

CHAPTER SIX

KEY #6—A HEALTH-PROMOTING DIET

STEP 1.
Reduce your fat intake

STEP 2.
Eat five or more servings of vegetables and fruits daily

STEP 3.
Limit your refined sugar intake

STEP 4.
Increase your fiber and complex carbohydrate intake

STEP 5.
Maintain protein intake at moderate levels

STEP 6.
Limit your salt intake

STEP 7.
Take time for meal planning

KEY #6—A HEALTH-PROMOTING DIET

It is now a well-established fact that certain dietary practices cause, while others prevent, a wide range of diseases. The evidence supporting diet's role in chronic degenerative diseases (including heart disease, cancer, stroke, diabetes, and arthritis) is substantial. Two basic facts support this link:

1. A diet rich in plant foods—whole grains, legumes, fruits, and vegetables—is protective against many diseases which are extremely common in Western society; and

2. A diet low in plant foods contributes to the development of these diseases, providing conditions under which other causative factors are more active.

The table below lists diseases with convincing links to a diet low in plant foods. Many of these diseases, which are quite common now, were extremely rare before the 20th century.

Diseases highly associated with a diet low in plant foods

Metabolic
Obesity, gout, diabetes, kidney stones, gallstones

Cardiovascular
Heart disease, high blood pressure, stroke, varicose veins, deep vein thrombosis, pulmonary embolism

Colonic
Constipation, appendicitis, diverticulitis, diverticulosis, hemorrhoids, colon cancer, irritable bowel syndrome, ulcerative colitis, Crohn's disease

Other
Dental caries, autoimmune disorders (such as rheumatoid arthritis), pernicious anemia, multiple sclerosis, eczema, thyrotoxicosis (toxicity due to an overactive thyroid gland)

Population studies, as well as clinical and experimental data, have proven these links. In 1984, the National Research Council's Food and Nutrition Board established the Committee on Diet and Health to undertake a comprehensive analysis of diet and major chronic diseases. (The Food and Nutrition Board develops the Recommended Dietary Allowance guidelines on the desirable amounts of essential nutrients in the diet.) Their findings, as well as those of the U.S. Surgeon General and highly respected medical groups, clearly show that Americans must change their eating habits to reduce their risk for chronic disease.

Trends in U.S. food consumption

There is little debate that a healthy diet must be rich in whole, natural and unprocessed foods. Fruits, vegetables, grains, beans, seeds and nuts are especially important. These foods contain not only valuable nutrients, but also dietary fiber and other compounds which have remarkable health-promoting properties.

Unfortunately, the modern Western diet presents quite a different picture. During this century, food consumption patterns have changed dramatically. Note the following:

- Total dietary fat intake has increased from 32% of daily calories to 43%.
- Overall carbohydrate intake has dropped from 57% to 46%.
- Protein intake has remained fairly stable at about 11%.

Compounding these detrimental changes are the individual food choices accounting for them. These are detailed in the chart on page 74. Notice that we are consuming more meat, fats, oils, sugars and sweeteners while we are eating less non-citrus fruits, vegetables, potatoes, and grain products. These changes have resulted in a drop in the percentage of calories from starches or complex carbohydrates, as found naturally occurring in grains and vegetables, from 68% in 1909 to 47% in 1980.

Currently, more than half of the carbohydrates we eat are in the form of refined sugars (sucrose, corn syrup, etc.) which are added to foods as sweetening agents. High consumption of refined sugars is linked to many chronic diseases, including obesity, diabetes, heart disease, and cancer.

Trends in quantities of foods consumed per capita (lb/year)

FOODS	1909—1913	1967—1969	1985
MEAT, POULTRY, AND FISH			
Beef	54	81	79
Pork	62	61	62
Poultry	18	46	70
Fish	12	15	19
Total	*146*	*203*	*230*
EGGS	37	40	32
DAIRY PRODUCTS			
Whole milk	223	232	122
Low-fat milk	64	44	112
Cheese	5	15	26
Other	28	100	86
Total	*320*	*391*	*346*
FATS AND OILS			
Butter	18	6	5
Margarine	1	10	11
Shortening	8	16	23
Lard and beef tallow	12	5	4
Salad and cooking oil	2	16	25
Total	*41*	*54*	*67*
FRUITS			
Citrus	17	60	72
Non-citrus, fresh	154	73	87
Non-citrus, processed	8	35	34
Total	*179*	*168*	*193*
VEGETABLES			
Tomatoes	46	36	38
Dark green and yellow	34	25	31
Other, fresh	136	87	96
Other, processed	11	35	29
Total	*227*	*183*	*194*
POTATOES, WHITE			
Fresh	182	67	55
Processed	0	15	28
Total	*182*	*82*	*83*
DRY BEANS, PEAS, NUTS, AND SOYBEANS	16	16	18
GRAIN PRODUCTS			
Wheat products	216	116	122
Corn products	56	15	7
Other grains	19	13	26
Total	*291*	*144*	*155*
SUGAR AND SWEETENERS			
Refined sugar	77	100	63
Syrups and other sweeteners	14	22	90
Total	*91*	*122*	*153*
MISCELLANEOUS	10	17	14

Source: National Research Council, *Diet and Health: Implications for Reducing Chronic Disease Risk* (Washington, DC, National Academy Press, 1989).

The government and nutrition education

Throughout the years, various governmental organizations have published dietary guidelines, but the recommendations of the United States Department of Agriculture (USDA) have become the most widely known. In 1956, the USDA published "Food for Fitness—A Daily Food Guide," which became popularly known as the Basic Four Food Groups. The Basic Four was composed of:

1. The Milk Group—milk, cheese, ice cream, and other milk-based foods.
2. The Meat Group—meat, fish, poultry, eggs, with dried legumes and nuts as alternatives.
3. The Fruit and Vegetable Group.
4. The Breads and Cereals Group.

One of the major problems with this model is that it graphically suggests all four food groups are equal in health value. The result? Overconsumption of animal products, dietary fat, and refined carbohydrates, and insufficient consumption of fiber-rich foods like fruits, vegetables, and legumes. This dietary imbalance is responsible for many premature deaths, chronic diseases, and increased health care costs. According to the U.S. Surgeon General's Report on Nutrition and Health, diet-related diseases account for 68% of all deaths in this country.

As the Basic Four Food Groups became outdated, various other governmental and medical organizations developed guidelines of their own. These were designed to either reduce a specific chronic degenerative disease (like cancer or heart disease) or reduce the risk for all chronic diseases. The recommendations of the U.S. Surgeon General, U.S. Senate, U.S. Department of Health and Human Services, American Heart Association, National Cancer Institute, American Diabetes Association, and the National Research Council's Committee on Diet and Health are all remarkably similar to the recommendations I am making.

Quite simply, a health-promoting diet provides optimal levels of all known nutrients and low levels of food components which are detrimental to health, such as sugar, saturated fats, cholesterol, salt, and food additives. A health-promoting diet is rich in whole "natural" and unprocessed foods. It is especially high in plant foods, such as fruits, vegetables, grains, beans, seeds and nuts, as these foods contain valuable nutrients and a variety of other compounds with remarkable health-promoting properties.

STEP 1. *Reduce your fat intake*

Current recommendations are that total fat intake be less than 30% of calories, with less than 10% of calories coming from saturated fat, and that the intake of cholesterol be less than 300 mg daily. The easiest way to achieve these recommendations is to limit your intake of animal products and not to use butter, margarine, salad dressings, gravy, creamy sauces, and other high-fat foods.

STEP 2. *Eat five or more servings of vegetables and fruits daily*

Fruits and vegetables are rich in fiber, vitamins, minerals, antioxidants and dozens of recently discovered phytochemicals which protect our body cells from damage. A high intake of fruits and vegetables has been shown to help protect against aging, cancer, heart disease, and many other degenerative conditions. Despite the well-known health benefits of frequent fruit and vegetable intake, fewer than 10% of all Americans eat the recommended quantity of five or more servings daily.

STEP 3. *Limit your refined sugar intake*

Carbohydrates provide us with the energy we need for body functions. There are two groups of carbohydrates, simple and complex. Simple carbohydrates, or sugars, are quickly absorbed by the body for a ready source of energy. The assortment of natural simple sugars in plant foods has an advantage over sucrose (white sugar) and other refined sugars because they are balanced by fiber and a wide range of nutrients. Problems with carbohydrates begin when they are refined and stripped of these nutrients. Virtually all of the vitamin content has been removed from white sugar, white breads and pastries, and many breakfast cereals. When high-sugar foods are eaten alone, the blood sugar level rises quickly, producing a strain on blood sugar control. Sources of refined sugar should be limited. Read food labels carefully for clues on sugar content. If the words sucrose, glucose, maltose, lactose, fructose, corn syrup, or white grape juice concentrate appear on the label, extra sugar has been added.

Refined carbohydrates are known to contribute to problems in blood sugar control, especially hypoglycemia (low blood sugar). When glucose levels are low, as occurs during hypoglycemia, the brain does not function properly. Such malfunction can result in anxiety, dizziness, headache, clouding of vision, blunted mental acuity, emotional instability, confusion, and abnormal behavior.

The association between hypoglycemia and impaired mental function is well known. Unfortunately, most individuals experiencing depression, anxiety, or other psychological conditions are rarely tested for hypoglycemia nor are they prescribed a diet which restricts refined carbohydrates.

STEP 4. *Increase your fiber and complex carbohydrate intake*

While refined carbohydrates should be restricted, the intake of complex carbohydrates should be increased. Complex carbohydrates, or starches, are composed of many simple sugars (polysaccharides) joined together by chemical bonds. The body breaks these bonds, releasing the simple sugars gradually, which leads to better blood sugar control. More and more research is indicating that complex carbohydrates should form a major part of the diet. Vegetables, legumes, and grains are excellent sources of complex carbohydrates.

In addition, these foods are excellent sources of dietary fiber. The term "dietary fiber" refers to the components of plant cell walls as well as the indigestible residues of plant foods. It is well established that a fiber-deficient diet is an important factor in the development of many chronic degenerative diseases.

Beneficial effects of dietary fiber

- Decreased intestinal transit time
- Delayed gastric emptying, resulting in reduced after-meal elevations of blood sugar
- Decreased caloric intake and appetite
- Increased pancreatic secretion, providing more digestive enzymes
- Increased stool weight
- More advantageous intestinal microflora
- Decreased cholesterol and triglyceride levels
- More soluble bile which improves absorption of fat-soluble vitamins

Step 5. *Maintain protein intake at moderate levels*

After water, protein is the next most plentiful component of our body. The body manufactures proteins to make up hair, muscles, nails, tendons, ligaments, and other body structures. Proteins also function as enzymes, hormones, and as important components of other cells such as our genes. Adequate protein intake is essential to good health, but too much protein causes problems.

One of the key recommendations of the National Research Council's Committee on Diet and Health was that Americans need to reduce protein intake to moderate levels. Americans consume much more protein than is required. Excess protein intake has been linked to several chronic diseases including cancer, osteoporosis, kidney disease, and heart disease. Reducing protein intake is best done by reducing meat and dairy consumption. Limit your intake to no more than 4 to 6 ounces per day and choose fish or skinless poultry. When you do eat meat, choose lean cuts rather than fat-laden choices.

STEP 6. *Limit your salt intake*

The balance of sodium to potassium is extremely important to human health. Too much sodium in the diet can disrupt this balance. In our society, only 5% of sodium intake comes from the natural ingredients in food. Prepared foods contribute 45% of our sodium intake, 45% is added in cooking, and another 5% is added as a condiment. Excessive consumption of dietary sodium chloride (table salt), coupled with diminished dietary potassium from fruits and vegetables, plays a major role in the development of cancer and cardiovascular disease (heart disease, high blood pressure, strokes, etc.). Conversely, a diet high in potassium and low in sodium is protective against these diseases, and, in the case of high blood pressure, can be therapeutic. To reduce your intake of sodium:

- Learn to enjoy the unsalted flavor of foods.
- Cook with only small amounts of salt and use flavor-enhancing herbs and "salt substitutes."
- Limit your intake of heavily salted foods like potato chips, pretzels, cheese, pickled foods, and cured meats.
- Read food labels carefully and avoid highly salted prepared or packaged foods.

STEP 7. *Take time for menu planning*

Most Americans do not take any time to think about menu planning. Instead they find themselves in a rush and often resort to eating out at a "fast-food" restaurant or skipping a meal. Both practices can have a negative effect on health. Take a few minutes each evening to plan out the next day's menu. Or, if you can do it, plan out a menu for the week. You'll more than recoup the time because you'll shop more efficiently and won't find yourself missing some ingredient for the night's meal. In addition, you'll likely save money since less browsing makes it easier to avoid impulse buys. Here are some healthful menu suggestions.

Breakfast

Time and again, studies have shown that people who eat breakfast weigh less, have more energy, and enjoy better health. Healthy breakfast choices include whole grain cereals, muffins, and breads along with fresh whole fruit or fresh fruit juice. Cereals, both hot and cold, preferably from whole grains, may be the best choices. Not only do the complex carbohydrates in the grains provide sustained energy, but an evaluation of data obtained from the National Health and Nutrition Examination Survey II (a survey of the nutritional and health practices of Americans) showed that serum cholesterol levels were lowest among adults eating whole grain cereal for breakfast. Although those individuals who consumed other breakfast foods had higher blood cholesterol levels, levels were highest among those who typically skipped breakfast.

Lunch

Lunch is a great time to enjoy a healthful bowl of soup, a large salad, and some whole grain bread. Due to their ability to improve blood sugar regulation, bean soups and other legume dishes are especially good lunch selections for people with diabetes and blood sugar problems. Beans and legumes are an excellent source of protein and fiber, yet are low in fat and calories.

Snacks

The best snacks are a handful of nuts or seeds, and some fresh fruit and vegetables (including fresh fruit and vegetable juice).

Dinner

For dinner, the healthiest meals include a fresh vegetable salad, a cooked vegetable side dish or bowl of soup, some whole grains, and legumes. The whole grains may be provided in bread, pasta, as a side dish, or as part of the recipe for an entree. The legumes can be utilized in soups, salads, and entrees.

Although a varied diet rich in whole grains, vegetables and legumes can provide optimal levels of protein, many people like to eat meat. The important thing is not to overconsume animal products. Again, limit your intake to no more than 4 to 6 ounces per day and choose fish or skinless poultry. When you do eat red meat, opt for lean cuts rather than fat-laden choices.

CHAPTER SEVEN

KEY #7—SUPPLEMENTATION

STEP 1.
Take a high-potency multiple vitamin and mineral formula

STEP 2.
Take additional antioxidants

STEP 3.
Use formulas designed to support specific body functions

STEP 4.
Use glandular support

STEP 5.
Use purified, standardized botanical extracts

STEP 6.
Use homeopathic remedies

STEP 7.
Use natural medicines

KEY #7—SUPPLEMENTATION

"Enzymatic therapy" is the final key to vibrant health. What is enzymatic therapy? Each type of enzyme in your body depends on nutrients to function at peak levels. When you selectively use nutrients to support these enzymes, you're using "enzymatic therapy."

Of course, Enzymatic Therapy is also the name of the company I founded. Enzymatic Therapy, the company, designs nutritional and herbal products for specific body functions. Different body tissues are made up of different enzymes and, therefore, have different needs. That's why Enzymatic Therapy has developed specific nutritional formulas for the bones, joints, heart and circulation, vision, liver, the thymus gland, gum health, and many, many more. We have more than 180 nutritional products to address your unique nutritional profile.

What are enzymes?

Enzymes are molecules that speed up the chemical reactions in your body. Without enzymes, these reactions would proceed too slowly to be useful to the body. Enzymes work by making or breaking chemical bonds, either joining molecules together or splitting them apart. Each enzyme affects a different chemical reaction.

Most of the enzymes in your body are composed of a protein and an essential mineral. If an enzyme is lacking its essential mineral, it can't function properly. It needs "enzymatic therapy." When you provide the necessary mineral through diet or supplementation, you allow the enzyme to perform its vital function.

For example, the enzyme that activates vitamin A in your visual process requires zinc. Without zinc, the enzyme can't convert vitamin A to its active form. In other words, if you're not getting enough zinc, you could face night blindness. However, when you boost your intake of zinc, you are using "enzymatic therapy" to allow the enzyme to fulfill its function.

Enzymes need coenzymes; coenzymes need nutrients

Most of the enzymes in your body rely on coenzymes, molecules that work cooperatively with the enzymes. Coenzymes are typically made up of vitamins and/or minerals. Without the proper coenzyme, an enzyme is powerless.

For example, vitamin C is a coenzyme to proline hydroxylase, an enzyme involved in collagen development. Collagen is the primary substance in connective tissue, cartilage, and bone. A vitamin C deficiency could sabotage collagen formation. Symptoms of this impairment would include poor wound healing, bleeding gums, and easy bruising. You could have plenty of proline hydroxylase in your system, but it can't do the job without vitamin C, its coenzyme and ally.

Providing enzymatic therapy through supplements

Enzymatic therapy involves the use of vitamins, minerals, enzymes, glandular concentrates, botanical extracts, and other natural compounds that work with the body's enzymes. As I mentioned before, specific body tissues are made up of specific enzymes, which depend on specific nutrients. During certain times—when you're under a lot of stress, for example—these nutritional needs may be magnified. And that's where supplements can help.

Over the past several years, more Americans than ever are discovering the advantages of nutritional and herbal supplements. However, medical experts have been slow to accept their value, despite the overwhelming scientific evidence that supports it.

In the world of nutrition and health, there are at least two distinct "camps." Some insist that diet alone can provide all the nutrition we need. Others tout the health benefits of supplemental vitamins and minerals. And you may feel like you're caught in the middle, trying to figure out which side is right.

To some extent, both sides are right. What it all boils down to is whether we're talking about minimum nutrition or optimum nutrition. If you simply want to avoid any obvious signs of nutritional deficiency, a balanced diet may be enough. However, if you're seeking optimal nutrition that allows you to function with the highest possible degree of vitality, enthusiasm, and passion for living, you may need something more.

Do you believe health is simply the absence of sickness? Or do you believe health is much more? The World Health Organization (WHO) defines health as "a state of complete physical, mental, and social well-being, not merely the absence of disease or infirmity." It's this goal of optimal, vibrant health that compels people to take nutritional and herbal supplements.

Why you may need supplements

If you're like most Americans, you probably aren't getting enough of all the nutrients you need. You may not suffer from any glaring nutritional deficiencies, but you could have a "subclinical" or marginal deficiency—a shortage of a particular vitamin or mineral that isn't severe enough to produce an obvious deficiency symptom.

The symptoms of subclinical deficiencies are often quite vague. You may feel fatigued or lethargic. You may find it difficult to concentrate. Or you may notice a general lack of well-being. Diagnosing subclinical deficiencies correctly is a complex process that involves detailed dietary or laboratory analysis.

Plenty of solid evidence shows that subclinical nutritional deficiencies are quite common. In recent years, the United States government has sponsored a number of comprehensive studies such as HANES I and II, the Ten State Nutrition Survey, and USDA nationwide food consumption research. These studies revealed marginal nutritional deficiencies in about 50%—that's half!—the population. In addition, over 80% of individuals in certain age groups consumed less than the RDA for specific nutrients.

What does this tell you? The chances are extremely slim that you can meet the Recommended Dietary Allowances (RDAs) for all nutrients by following the typical American diet. Yes, it is theoretically possible for a healthy individual to get all the necessary nutrition through food. But the reality is, most Americans do not even come close to eating a completely nutritious diet.

Is the RDA enough?

Most people have probably heard of RDAs due to recent changes in nutritional labeling. But what are RDAs exactly? And how do they relate to our level of nutrition and health?

Since 1941, the Food and Nutrition Board of the National Research Council has prepared RDAs for vitamins and minerals. These guidelines were originally developed to reduce the rates of severe nutritional deficiencies such as scurvy (deficiency of vitamin C), pellagra (deficiency of niacin), and beriberi (deficiency of vitamin B1). Furthermore, the RDAs were designed with large population groups in mind—not individuals. However, we know that each person has distinct and unique nutritional requirements. Even the Food and Nutrition Board concedes that "Individuals with special nutritional needs are not covered by the RDAs."

RDAs focus only on preventing obvious nutritional deficiencies in specific population groups. They do not define optimal intake for an individual. A tremendous amount of scientific research tells us that the optimal level for many nutrients—especially the antioxidants—may be much higher than their RDA.

RDAs also don't consider environmental and lifestyle factors that can destroy vitamins and bind minerals. For example, the Food and Nutrition Board admits that smokers require at least twice as much vitamin C as non-smokers. Of course, this raises further questions: What about the impact of smoking on other nutrients? What about the effects of alcohol, food additives, pesticides, heavy metals (lead, mercury, etc.), carbon monoxide, and other chemicals that are a part of our society? How do these factors interfere with our nutritional status?

The RDAs have done an excellent job of defining what we need to prevent severe nutritional deficiencies. But we still have a great deal to learn about optimal nutrition. RDAs can help us avoid deficiency diseases, but optimal nutrition can help us truly thrive.

STEP 1. *Take a high-potency multiple vitamin and mineral formula*
Building optimal health requires a strong foundation. A balanced, high-potency vitamin and mineral supplement is an essential part of that foundation. As I mentioned before, it's difficult to get all the vitamins and minerals our bodies need through diet alone—especially if we're trying to improve our health. A high-potency multiple formula can provide solid nutritional insurance.

If you've looked at all the multiple formulas available, you may have felt overwhelmed by the choices. How do you know what to look for? What's the best combination of nutrients for your particular body and lifestyle?

First, when you're shopping for a multiple formula, make sure it provides a full range of vitamins and minerals.

Vitamins
Each of the 13 known vitamins has its own special role to play. They fall into two groups: fat-soluble (A, D, E, and K) and water-soluble (the B vitamins and vitamin C). Vitamins work with enzymes in the chemical reactions necessary for bodily functions, including energy production.

Minerals

Twenty-two different minerals are also important for human nutrition: boron, calcium, chloride, chromium, cobalt, copper, fluoride, germanium, iodide, iron, magnesium, manganese, molybdenum, phosphorous, potassium, selenium, silicon, sodium, sulfur, tin, vanadium, and zinc.

Second, be aware that men and women have different nutritional needs. Make sure the multiple formula you choose provides extra amounts of the specific vitamins and minerals that your body may require.

Nutrition for men

Nutrients especially important for men include niacin, magnesium, and zinc. Niacin and magnesium are essential for cardiovascular function. Cardiovascular health is a big concern for most men, and for good reason. In a 26-year follow-up of more than 5,000 people involved in the Framingham Heart Study, the rate of heart disease in men age 35 to 44 was more than six times greater than in women of the same age.

Zinc is important for the male sex glands. Testosterone synthesis and activity, sperm development, and prostate function all rely on proper levels of zinc. In fact, the highest concentration of zinc in a man's body is located in the prostate.

Specific herbs may also be useful for male health. Muira puama (also known as potency wood) is highly regarded in Brazil. Korean ginseng, the most famous plant in China, is often used alone or in combination with other herbs for the male system. The liposterolic extract of the saw palmetto berry contains fatty acids and sterols, important factors for the prostate gland.

Nutrition for women

Nutrients especially important for women include calcium, iron, and vitamin B6. Calcium and iron deficiencies are common among women, and vitamin B6 is involved in some of the hormonal processes of the menstrual cycle.

In addition, women have depended on a variety of herbs throughout the centuries, such as dong quai, chaste berry, and fennel seed. In Asia, dong quai is recognized as a "female plant," and its reputation is second only to ginseng. Chaste berry, which grows in the

Mediterranean region, is popular in Europe. The Kommission E of the German Health Authority recommends this herb to menstruating women. And fennel seed contains phytoestrogens (natural plant estrogens) and other natural compounds linked to female health.

Choose a supplement targeted to your needs

With this information in mind, it's easy to see why Enzymatic Therapy created **Doctor's Choice**™ **for Men** and **Doctor's Choice for Women**™. Michael T. Murray, N.D., our Director of Research and one of the world's leading authorities on natural medicine and supplements, designed these formulas to provide optimal nutrition for the male and female systems.

Based on his in-depth research and extensive nutritional knowledge, Dr. Murray has prepared just the right blend of essential nutrients and botanical extracts for men and women. He has included all the key vitamins, minerals, and herbs in their most beneficial amounts. That's why I recommend these two daily multiples for anyone who wants to build a strong nutritional foundation. For general nutritional support, take one tablet three times daily with meals; for extra support, you may take two or three tablets with meals.

STEP 2. *Take additional antioxidants*

You've probably heard about the importance of antioxidants such as vitamin C, vitamin E, selenium, and beta-carotene. Antioxidants protect your cells from the damaging effects of compounds known as free radicals or pro-oxidants. Unfortunately, your cells are constantly attacked by these highly reactive molecules, which can bind to and destroy parts of the cell.

Free radicals are produced in the body during normal metabolic processes such as energy production, detoxification, and immune mechanisms. Lifestyle and environment may also contribute to your free-radical burden. For example, cigarette smoke greatly increases the level of free radicals in your body which, in turn, depletes the level of vitamin C and beta-carotene. This depletion leaves the cells—especially the ones lining your airways—unprotected and susceptible to damage.

Other external sources of free radicals include ionizing radiation, chemotherapeutic drugs, anesthetics, air pollutants, pesticides, fried foods, alcohol, solvents, and formaldehyde. These toxic substances greatly burden the body's defense mechanisms. If you're exposed to these factors, you should consider getting additional antioxidant support.

How the body handles free radicals

Free radicals can't cause damage once they are broken down or chemically neutralized. To protect itself, your body produces its own free-radical-scavenging enzymes such as catalase, superoxide dismutase (SOD), and glutathione peroxidase. However, research shows that taking these antioxidant enzymes in supplement form won't increase their levels in the body. What you can do is increase your intake of their nutritional cofactors. For example, adding supplemental manganese to your diet can help increase SOD concentrations in your body.

On the other hand, you can increase your tissue levels of specific antioxidant nutrients directly through diet or supplementation. Antioxidants such as beta-carotene, vitamins C and E, and selenium help protect your cells by binding to free radicals and neutralizing them.

A complete "Cellular Protection System"

A well-rounded antioxidant product should include all the important antioxidants plus the nutrient cofactors needed for free-radical-scavenging enzymes. That's why Dr. Murray developed **CPS** (Cellular Protection System) for Enzymatic Therapy. This super-antioxidant formula nourishes all parts of your cells to protect them inside and out. It provides beta carotene, vitamin C, vitamin E, manganese, selenium, and zinc. It also has riboflavin, which helps regenerate antioxidants after they have neutralized free radicals.

What sets CPS apart from other antioxidant formulas? It contains several other compounds with potent antioxidant activity: flavonoids extracted from grape seeds and green tea, curcumin (the yellow pigment of turmeric), and N-acetylcysteine (a stable form of the essential amino acid cysteine). CPS also provides concentrated extracts of cabbage, garlic, ginger, and Klamath blue-green algae. These foods contain a broad range of antioxidants. Cabbage, for example, is a good source of powerful sulfur-containing compounds such as thiols, indoles, and isothiocyanates. These compounds not only protect cells, they also support the body's detoxification processes. In fact, the American Cancer Society has recommended that Americans increase their intake of cabbage-family vegetables because of their health-promoting features.

The whole CPS formula is greater than the sum of its individual parts. One or two capsules with meals will help saturate your tissues with free-radical-scavenging antioxidants.

The power of herbal antioxidants

Research shows that certain herbal flavonoids are "tissue-specific antioxidants." This means they target specific areas of the body. Here are just a few of the links researchers have noted:

Flavonoid source	*Specific target*
Bilberry	Eyes
Silymarin from milk thistle	Liver
Ginkgo	Brain, lining of the arteries
Hawthorn	Heart
Grape seed	Lining of the blood vessels

When a specific body tissue requires additional antioxidant support, natural health care professionals will often recommend the appropriate plant extract.

Grape seed extract is an especially potent source of antioxidant protection. Grape seed extract contains flavonoid compounds called procyanidolic oligomers (PCOs), which have 20 to 50 times more antioxidant activity than vitamins C and E. Although PCOs can also come from pine bark extract, studies show that grape seed extract contains higher amounts of PCOs. And, only grape seed extract contains the gallic esters of proanthocyanidins, the most active free-radical scavengers known.

At Enzymatic Therapy, we combined grape seed extract with phosphatidylcholine to produce **Grape Seed (PCO) Phytosome®**. Phosphatidylcholine, a natural component of lecithin, acts as an emulsifier. The patented phytosome process binds phosphatidyl-choline to PCO molecules, creating new molecules that are absorbed and transported more efficiently in the body. This means more PCOs are delivered to body tissues. In fact, phytosome research indicates that herbal compounds bound to phosphatidylcholine are three to seven times more bioavailable than unbound compounds.

As you can see, there's much more to antioxidants than just beta carotene and vitamin C. Nature provides a wide range of powerful compounds to help protect your cells.

STEP 3. *Use formulas designed to support specific body functions*

Years of study and experience have shown that specific vitamins, minerals, herbs, and glandular concentrates produce far better dietary results when combined than when taken individually. Enzymatic Therapy carved its niche in the nutritional supplement industry by developing specific combinations of these natural substances to support specific body functions. To give you an example of how one of our formulas targets a certain body tissue, let's look at **Liv-A-Tox**. This product provides nutrients essential for liver function.

Example: specific nutrients for the liver

The liver is truly a remarkable organ. As the largest gland in your body, it participates in metabolism, the process that breaks down the food you eat into nutrients and energy. It detoxifies harmful compounds such as drugs, pesticides, poisons, and excess cholesterol. It filters the blood, removing bacteria, dead cells, and waste materials. It produces and secretes bile to help you digest and absorb fats. It stores iron, vitamins, and glycogen. And it is the only gland in your body that can regenerate itself.

Because the liver is so vitally important, Enzymatic Therapy developed Liv-A-Tox. This supplement combines the following ingredients:

- Essential vitamins: A, B12, C, niacin, biotin. The antioxidant vitamins A and C assist the liver's detoxifying mechanisms. In fact, the liver stores most of the body's vitamin A—about 90%. The liver also stores large quantities of B vitamins (including B12, niacin and biotin) needed for the proper synthesis of enzymes involved in carbohydrate and fat metabolism.

- Lipotropic substances: Methionine, choline, vitamin B12. Lipotropic substances help the body break down fats and use them properly. Methionine, an essential amino acid, is the major lipotropic compound in the body. Methionine levels affect the amount of sulfur-containing compounds, such as glutathione, in the liver. Glutathione and other sulfur-containing peptides (small proteins) play a critical role in defending against toxic compounds. Choline, an integral part of cell membranes, and vitamin B12 also assist detoxification reactions in the liver.

- Herbal extracts: Green beet leaf powder, barberry, celandine, cheonanthus, boldo. These herbs have been used throughout history to support liver function. Modern research is showing that the natural compounds in these plants have significant benefit for the human body. For example, several clinical studies have shown a link between bile flow and berberine, an alkaloid compound in barberry.

- Other natural factors: Inositol, desiccated liver, unsaturated free fatty acids. Inositol, an important constituent of cell membranes, has shown lipotropic activity in various animal studies. Desiccated liver is a dried, powdered form of whole liver. Unsaturated free fatty acids play an essential role in the regulation of cholesterol metabolism.

Every nutrient we use in our formulas is backed by solid research, certified lab tested, and guaranteed to be of the highest quality.

Nutritional formulas offer long-term value

Nutritional formulas like Liv-A-Tox are not designed to treat diseases. They are not drugs. Instead of attacking isolated symptoms, they nourish your body, working with its natural processes. Although their influence is often gradual, their long-term benefit can be enormous. When you give your body the nutritional building blocks it needs, health improvements will often follow.

Step 4. *Use glandular support*

For almost as long as historic records have been kept, people have used glandular therapy. "Like helps like" is the basic concept underlying the use of glandular substances from animals. For example, if your adrenal glands need support, you may find value in supplementing your diet with a concentrated adrenal gland extract.

What is a gland?

A gland is defined as an organ that secretes something, usually hormones, into the bloodstream. The body's glands include: pineal, pituitary, thyroid, parathyroid, thymus, adrenal, pancreas, and gonads (testes or ovaries). Although they are not technically glands, other organs are often called "glandulars," too. Extracts of heart, spleen, prostate, uterus, brain, and other tissues are often used in glandular or organotherapy.

Most glandular products come from beef (bovine) sources. The exceptions are pancreatic enzymes, which are typically derived from pork (porcine) sources.

Are glandulars useful?

Science has confirmed that specific glandular preparations are useful when taken orally. Those containing active hormones or enzymes—such as thyroid, adrenal cortex, and pancreatin preparations—are particularly beneficial. In addition, a great deal of research supports the use of pharmaceutical-grade extracts of the liver, aorta, and thymus. There's also some support for pituitary, spleen, orchic (testes) and ovarian extracts.

Despite the scientific support, many people still question the value of glandular products for the human body. I believe it's not a question of health value; it's a question of product quality. What we really need to ask is whether most glandular supplements currently available have merit.

At this time, the glandular industry does not enforce strict quality control procedures or standards for these products. Individual companies must develop and enforce their own good manufacturing practices. And it all begins with how the raw material is processed.

To get full value from glandular supplements, the raw material must be prepared correctly to ensure that the biologically active compounds—the enzymes, soluble proteins, natural lipid factors, vitamins, minerals, and hormone precursors—are not destroyed or eliminated. The four most widely known methods of processing glandulars are: azeotrophic method, salt precipitation, freeze-drying, and predigesting. Let's look at these methods in more detail.

Azeotrophic method

This process begins by quick-freezing the material at a temperature well below 0° Fahrenheit. The material is then washed with a powerful solvent (ethylene dichloride) to remove fatty tissue. After the solvent is distilled off, the material is dried and ground into a powder, which is then placed in tablets or capsules.

Although the azeotrophic method eliminates fat-stored toxins such as pesticides and heavy metals, it also removes important fat-soluble hormones, enzymes, essential fatty acids, and other potentially valuable compounds. In addition, traces of the solvent remain in the final product.

Salt precipitation

The salt precipitation method breaks up fresh glandular material in salt and water. The salt increases the density of the water-soluble material. As a result, when the mixture is centrifuged, the lighter, fat-soluble material can be separated out. This material is then dried into a powder.

The benefit of salt precipitation is that no toxic solvent is used to separate the fatty material. The drawback, however, is that most people don't need the remaining salt.

Freeze-dried

In the freeze-drying process, the glandular material is quickly frozen at 40 to 60° below zero Fahrenheit. Then the frozen material is placed in a vacuum chamber, where the water is removed through direct vaporization—hence the term "freeze-dried." This low-temperature drying cycle ensures that the biologically active state of the gland's vitamins, enzymes, hormones, and natural cofactors remains intact.

Freeze-drying is advantageous because it produces a higher concentration of unaltered protein and enzymes with all of the important fat-soluble components. However, because the fat is not removed, the glands must come from livestock that grazed on open ranges where no pesticides or herbicides were used. The animals must also be free from exposure to antibiotics, synthetic hormones, and infection.

Predigestion

The predigestion process produces a soluble glandular concentrate that's more easily digested and better absorbed in the body. Predigestion uses plant and animal enzymes to partially digest or hydrolyze (break down) the glandular material. The partially digested material is passed through a series of filtrations to separate out fat-soluble and large molecules. The processed material is then freeze-dried. This method is especially ideal for glandulars such as liver and thymus concentrates, where the most valuable compounds are the polypeptide (small amino-acid chains) and other water-soluble fractions.

I feel that predigested soluble concentrates are the best. Like all foods, glandulars must be digested to extract their nutrients. Because predigested glandulars need little or no further digestion, the body can assimilate their natural factors quickly and easily. That's why most glandulars in Enzymatic Therapy products are predigested.

Enzymatic Therapy's glandular concentrates

Enzymatic Therapy's glandular concentrates come from healthy livestock range-fed in New Zealand, where ranchers use no herbicides, pesticides, hormones, or antibiotics. The glands and organs of these grass-fed animals are much higher in vitamins, carotene, and valuable biochemical factors than the glands and organs of grain-fed animals. EEC and USDA government inspectors thoroughly examine all the glands and organs we use and certify that they are free from disease, abnormality, and contamination.

For all these reasons, you can count on the quality and consistency of Enzymatic Therapy's glandular supplements.

STEP 5. *Use purified, standardized botanical extracts*

For many people in the world, herbal medicines are the only therapeutic agents available. In 1985, the World Health Organization estimated that 80% of the world's population relied on herbs for their primary health care needs.

In addition, 30 to 40% of all medical doctors in France and Germany rely on herbal preparations as their primary medicines. These physicians typically use herbal products that are standardized to contain a specific level of active compounds. In the United States, these products are known as Purified Standardized Extracts (P.S.E.s). Enzymatic Therapy was the first U.S. company to develop P.S.E.s (also known as "guaranteed potency extracts").

Before we discuss the value of P.S.E.s, let's look at how herbs are marketed in the United States compared to other parts of the world.

Herbal products around the world

Most herbal products cannot be marketed in the United States with any medical claims. In contrast, herbal products in Germany can be marketed with medical claims, as long as they have been proven safe and effective. In Germany, the legal requirements for herbal medicines are identical to those for all other drugs. Whether the herbal product is available by prescription or over-the-counter (OTC) depends on its application and safety. If prescribed by a physician, herbal products sold in pharmacies are covered by insurance.

To regulate the safety and quality of herbal preparations, the German Health Authority established a special panel of physicians, pharmacologists, and toxicologists. Called the "Kommission E," this expert panel developed a series of 200 monographs for herbal products similar to the OTC monographs for synthetic drugs prepared by the U.S. Food and Drug Administration (FDA). In Germany, an herbal product is viewed as safe and effective if a manufacturer meets the quality requirements of the monographs or provides additional evidence of safety and effectiveness. This proof can include data from existing literature, anecdotal information from practicing physicians, and limited clinical studies.

In the United States, herbs are classified as foods or food additives (that's why their labels can't list any medicinal uses or dosage information). To reach the status of an over-the-counter medicine, plants must go through a rigorous and costly testing process that usually lasts six to ten years. The process involves safety tests on animals and human volunteers, and complex efficacy tests on groups of healthy and ill patients. The FDA rarely approves a product based on existing literature, research done outside the United States, or anecdotal evidence.

Ginkgo biloba provides an excellent example of the differences in these regulatory approaches. In Germany and France, extracts of Ginkgo biloba leaves are registered for the treatment of cerebral and peripheral vascular insufficiency (reduced blood flow to the brain and extremities). Available by prescription and over the counter, ginkgo extracts are among the top three most widely prescribed medicines in Germany and France, with combined annual sales of more than $500 million.

In contrast, Ginkgo biloba extracts identical to those approved in Germany and France are labeled "food supplements" in the United States. It would cost roughly $500 million to get the FDA to approve ginkgo as a medicinal product. However, a natural product can't be patented, so it doesn't have the same degree of marketing protection as a synthetic drug. It is simply not feasible for a company to spend that kind of money to get approval, when another company could then market the same product without spending a dime.

Unfortunately, the FDA has rejected the idea of establishing an independent advisory panel to develop herbal monographs similar to Germany's Kommission E monographs. They have also dismissed other ideas to create an appropriate framework for the marketing of herbal products in the United States.

Forms of herbal preparations

Commercial herbal preparations are available in several different forms: bulk herbs, teas, tinctures, fluid extracts, and tablets or capsules. It is important for consumers, physicians, pharmacists, health food store personnel, and anyone else who routinely uses or recommends herbs to understand the differences among these forms.

Teas

When an herbal tea bag is steeped in hot water, it's actually a type of herbal extract called an infusion. The water acts as a solvent by drawing out some of the medicinal properties of the herb. Teas are often better sources of bioavailable compounds than the powdered herb. However, teas are weaker than tinctures, fluid extracts, and solid extracts.

Tinctures

To make a tincture, the herb is soaked in an alcohol and water mixture for a specific amount of time. This soaking usually lasts from several hours to several days, although it can be much longer for some herbs. The solution is then pressed out, leaving the tincture.

Fluid extracts

Fluid extracts are more concentrated than tinctures. They are typically made from alcohol and water mixtures, although other solvents may be used, such as vinegar, glycerine, or propylene glycol. Low-temperature techniques such as vacuum distillation or counter-current filtration are then used to distill off some of the alcohol.

Solid extract

A solid extract is produced by further concentrating the herbal material through the mechanisms described for fluid extracts. The solvent is completely removed, leaving a viscous (soft) solid extract or a dry solid extract, depending on the herb, portion of the plant, and processing method used. If it's not already in powder form, the dry solid extract can be ground into coarse granules or a fine powder. A solid extract can also be diluted with alcohol and water to make a tincture or fluid extract.

Strengths of extracts

The potencies or strengths of herbal extracts can be expressed in two ways: by the level of their active components or in terms of concentration. Let's talk about concentration first.

Tinctures are usually a 1:5 or 1:10 concentration. In a 1:5 concentration, one part of the herb (in grams) is soaked in five parts liquid (in milliliters of volume). In other words, a tincture contains five times more solvent than herbal material. Fluid extracts contain more herbal material. They are usually concentrated at a 1:1 ratio—one part herb to one part liquid. Solid extracts are even more concentrated, at a typical ratio of 4:1. This means one part of the extract is equivalent to, or derived from, four parts of the crude herb. Some solid extracts are concentrated as high as 100:1, which means it would take almost 100 pounds of crude herb to equal the material in one pound of the extract.

As you can see, a 4:1 solid extract is four times stronger than an equal amount of fluid extract, and up to 40 times stronger than an equal amount of tincture—as long as they are produced from the same quality of herb.

Standardization for consistent quality

In the past, many of the important components of herbs were unknown, so the quality of extracts was difficult to determine. However, recent advances in extraction processes, along with improved analytical methods, have raised the standards of quality control.

Because manufacturing techniques and raw materials vary widely, concentrating an herbal extract is not always the most accurate way to measure its potency. By using a high-quality herb—one with an optimal level of its most important components—we can produce a more potent tea, tincture, fluid extract or solid extract. Standardization of the key components guarantees herbal products that provide consistent purity and quality.

Standardized herbal products are commonly used in Europe, and their use is becoming more widespread here in the United States. In a standardized product, the level of the key compound is the same from one capsule to the next. Recommendations for these extracts are based on the level of their most important compounds rather than their concentration or extract weight.

Here are some examples of European recommendations for standardized herbal products:

- *Vaccinium myrtillus* (bilberry)
  40 mg of anthocyanosides
- *Silybum marianum* (milk thistle)
  70 mg of silymarin
- *Centella asiatica* (Gotu kola)
  30 mg of triterpenic acids

Even though these herbs are standardized for their most important compounds, they still contain other valuable constituents. Mother Nature packaged various plant compounds together for a reason. These constituents work best when they work synergistically.

Many herbs contain compounds that enhance the advantages of their most important component. For example, several "inactive" components of *Piper methysticum* (kava) promote the absorption and activity of the most important compounds, kavalactones. The same is true for *Ginkgo biloba*, *Uva ursi* (bearberry), *Hydrastis canadensis* (goldenseal), and many other herbs.

Pharmaceutical companies often isolate the active constituents of certain plants and then synthesize them. But when these compounds are taken out of their natural environment, they lose much of their value. Enzymatic Therapy's Purified Standardized Extracts™ typically contain all of the plant's natural constituents, but are standardized for a consistent level of the most important ones.

Quality control in herbal products

Manufacturing standardized herbal products requires the latest analytical and processing techniques. Herbal technology has seen many advances in harvesting schedules, cultivation techniques, storage, activity, stability of important compounds, and product purity. All of these factors help ensure a higher quality final product. Yet there is one factor even more vital than these: **quality control**.

Quality control refers to the processes that ensure the quality or validity of a product. To manufacture herbal products that work, quality control is essential. Without it, you have no way of knowing that what's printed on the label is actually what's present in the product. At this time, however, no organization or government agency monitors the quality of herbal products or the accuracy of their labels.

Unfortunately, this lack of quality control has tarnished the reputation of many important medicinal herbs. For example, about half of the *Echinacea purpurea* sold in the United States from 1908 through 1991 was actually *Parthenium integrifolium*, due to errors made in collecting the herb. Why did this happen? Both herbs are known as "Missouri snakeroot," and they look somewhat similar. But they are different species containing different compounds.

How do we solve this quality control problem? Manufacturers and suppliers of herbal products must follow strict quality control standards and good manufacturing practices. Laboratory analysis is now sophisticated enough to accurately identify plants, so we should—at the very least—be guaranteed that we're getting the herb we're paying for.

To promote higher quality control standards, consumers, health food stores, pharmacists, and physicians should ask for information about the herbal products they use and recommend. Do the manufacturers guarantee the validity of their herbal supplements? Are all their raw plant materials and final products laboratory tested? Are they standardized for a consistent level of their key compounds?

At Enzymatic Therapy, we have "self-imposed" the highest possible standards. Our Purified Standardized Extracts™ serve as a model of quality control for all forms of herbal preparations. Each batch of a particular extract is meticulously analyzed. We use microscopic evaluation, physical tests, and sophisticated chemical analysis to examine the product. It doesn't leave our facility unless it contains the proper ratio of important plant compounds and meets all of our strict quality control standards.

EchinaFresh™: An example of exceptional quality

An excellent example of our devotion to quality control is our fresh-pressed echinacea product, EchinaFresh. Produced in Switzerland, EchinaFresh contains the pure, fresh-pressed juice of the Echinacea purpurea plant. The echinacea we use is Certified Organic—a difficult certification to obtain in Switzerland—meaning that absolutely no pesticides and no chemical fertilizers are ever used. This echinacea is harvested only while in full bloom, when it's richest in natural compounds, and fresh-pressed immediately to capture its fullest potential. Only the stems, leaves, and flowers are used because they are more easily absorbed by the body.

EchinaFresh is available as a concentrated powdered extract in capsules and as a liquid. EchinaFresh capsules contain 50 milligrams of extract concentrated at a 50-to-1 ratio. This means it takes 50 pounds of fresh plants to make one pound of extract, so each capsule equals 2,500 milligrams of crude echinacea powder. EchinaFresh liquid contains two-thirds less alcohol than many other liquid echinacea products. After the echinacea is harvested and juiced, a small amount of alcohol is added to stabilize the quality.

EchinaFresh is the only echinacea product in the United States that provides a standardized content of beta-1,2-D-fructofuranosides. Fructofuranosides are sensitive biomarkers that reflect the level of freshness, purity, and potency. This product meets the German Kommission E monograph for echinacea, and every batch is certified lab-tested.

Garlinase 4000™: *Lab tests prove that what we claim is true*

Quality control also shines forth in our one-of-a-kind garlic supplement, Garlinase 4000. The benefits of garlic are well known. Visit any health food store and you'll see many different garlic supplements, each one claiming to be the "best." However, the quality of these products varies tremendously. Let's examine why.

The majority of garlic's benefits are clearly due to a compound called allicin. Unfortunately, allicin is also responsible for garlic's characteristic odor. To avoid this problem and still get the benefits of garlic, many companies have developed techniques that produce "odorless" garlic products.

An intact garlic bulb doesn't have much odor, because allicin doesn't exist in raw garlic. However, when garlic is cut or crushed, an enzyme called alliinase converts a compound called alliin into allicin. Products concentrated for alliin and other sulfur components provide all the benefits of fresh garlic, but are more "socially acceptable." These products are prepared in a way that allows the allicin to be formed once the tablet is inside the small intestine.

Manufacturers of such products often claim a very high "total allicin potential." Basically, this means the product has the "potential" to deliver high amounts of allicin but may not be stable, so the manufacturer can't guarantee the level of allicin at the most critical time—when the product is used. To provide maximum benefits, a garlic supplement must not only be standardized for its alliin content; it must also be stable.

What about aged garlic extracts? The German Kommission E monograph specifically recommends a daily intake equivalent to 4,000 mg of fresh, raw garlic (about 4 to 5 cloves). Since aged garlic preparations do not contain the beneficial compounds found in fresh garlic, they can't be marketed in Germany with the claims allowed for garlic. Manufacturers of aged garlic supplements tout the benefits of components other than allicin. However, you don't need to use an aged garlic preparation to get these components.

If you check the numbers, you will see that Garlinase 4000 is by far the most potent garlic product available. Other companies may make this claim, but only Enzymatic Therapy provides the proof. Each package of Garlinase 4000 comes with an independent laboratory analysis for the levels of alliin, alliinase, allicin and other beneficial compounds. Tests show that the levels of these compounds in Garlinase 4000 are actually higher than what is listed on the label. Lab analysis also confirms that Garlinase 4000 provides more gamma-glutamylcysteines (19,000 mcg per tablet) and precursors to ajoene and diallyldisulfides (6,000 mcg per tablet) than any other garlic product in the world, including aged garlic preparations.

In addition, Garlinase 4000 is the only garlic supplement available in America that delivers in just one tablet the full amount specified by the Kommission E monograph. Other companies may claim to have "one-per-day" products, but if they don't meet the Kommission E standard, is it right to make that claim?

When you purchase garlic or any other herbal supplement, look beyond the label claims. Look for the same level of analysis and documentation that Enzymatic Therapy provides with Garlinase 4000.

Step 6. *Use homeopathic medicines*

Homeopathy is a 200-year-old system of medicine in which symptoms are treated with minute quantities of drugs—usually herbs—that would normally cause those very same symptoms. Let's look at this more closely.

The word "homeopathy" comes from the Greek words *homoios*, which means like, and *pathos*, which means suffering. Homeopathy is based on the principle that "like cures like." In other words, a substance that can cause a symptom in a healthy person may treat that same symptom in a sick person. For example, when people cut into onions, their eyes water. A traditional homeopathic remedy for a cold or allergy sufferer with watery eyes would be a preparation of red onion.

The impact of homeopathic medicines is similar to that of vaccines. Unlike conventional medicines, homeopathic remedies don't attack the disease or condition. Instead, these highly diluted substances stimulate the body's own self-regulating and self-healing mechanisms. Basically, they help the body take care of its own symptoms.

Homeopathy was highly respected and widely used in the United States at the end of the 19th century, but as drug companies became more powerful, they effectively suppressed this effective and nontoxic form of medicine. However, homeopathy has remained popular in many other parts of the world (especially Europe and India), and is now making a strong comeback in the United States. Homeopathic medicines here are regulated by the FDA and must comply with the *Homeopathic Pharmacopoeia*.

Proven safe and effective

Homeopathy has been used very effectively for a variety of common ailments, both physical and mental. And scientific studies confirm that it works.

To illustrate the power of homeopathy, I want to tell you about a product called **Anti-Anxiety** from Lehning Laboratories, one of the leading manufacturers of homeopathic medicines in France since 1935. A clinical study compared Lehning's Anti-Anxiety to the drug diazepam in 60 women. Half received Anti-Anxiety; half received diazepam. Using the Hamilton scale (a scoring scale often used to assess anxiety), the patients were evaluated before and after a 30-day treatment.

Results showed that Anti-Anxiety was as effective as diazepam in reducing anxiety, phobia, and emotional instability. The same held true for symptoms that often accompany anxiety: hot flashes, rapid heartbeat, shortness of breath, intestinal problems, frequent urination, and dizziness. In addition, both groups experienced a significant increase in sleep and decrease in pulse rate.

The patients and physicians participating in this study agreed that Anti-Anxiety was as effective as diazepam in reducing symptoms of anxiety and depression. However, there are a few important differences. Diazepam can be severely toxic and addictive, but Anti-Anxiety has no side effects and is not habit-forming. It is also much less expensive.

I am proud that Enzymatic Therapy is the exclusive United States distributor of Anti-Anxiety and other Lehning products. Like Enzymatic Therapy, Lehning Laboratories is a family-owned company dedicated to producing the highest quality products of its kind. We carry a complete line of quality Lehning homeopathic remedies for common health problems such as acne, arthritis, asthma and allergies, bronchitis, cold and flu, fatigue (physical and mental), headaches, hemorrhoids, indigestion, insomnia, menopause, sinusitis, and more. We also offer several Lehning homeopathic products for children's health concerns such as colic, teething, nervous tension, sleeplessness, cold and flu symptoms, and allergies.

For more information

To learn more about homeopathy, I highly recommend a book entitled *Questions and Answers on Family Health* by Jan de Vries, Ph.D., one of the world's leading authorities on homeopathy. This book is available through IMPAKT Communications, Inc., for $10.95 (which includes shipping and handling). You may reach them at 1-800-477-2995, or use the order form at the back of this book.

Step 7. *Use natural medicines*

In many instances, you can find natural alternatives to synthetic over-the-counter medicines. OTC products can be used safely without medical supervision for symptoms that can be self-diagnosed. However, just because a product is available over-the-counter does not mean it's completely safe and nontoxic. Many OTC products have side effects ranging from mild discomfort to severe, health-threatening problems. For example, aspirin can irritate the stomach and cause bleeding and is known to interfere with blood clotting.

At Enzymatic Therapy, we search for natural over-the-counter medicines that provide relief with minimal or no side effects. Let's look at several examples.

Natural medicines for acne

Synthetic OTC acne products often contain benzoyl peroxide, which works by removing the top layer of the skin and killing bacteria. Too much benzoyl peroxide can dry the skin excessively, causing redness, peeling, and even blistering. Realizing this, Enzymatic Therapy developed the **Derma-Klear® Acne Treatment Program** using sulfur as the active ingredient. Sulfur helps fight the bacteria that causes acne with minimal drying of the skin and no burning or blistering. The Derma-Klear products also contain herbal extracts such as aloe vera, chamomile extract, and hawthorn extract.

The Derma-Klear Acne Treatment Program is one of the safest and most effective ways to treat and prevent acne. The natural cream, soap, and cleanser are hypoallergenic and contain no irritating fragrances, detergents, or chemicals. Best of all, they can be used in conjunction with Derma-Klear **Akne-Zyme**™, a nutritional supplement that supports healthy skin from the inside out. This comprehensive formula provides essential vitamins and minerals for the skin, such as vitamin A, vitamin C, the B vitamins, and zinc.

The Derma-Klear Acne Treatment Program is excellent for teenagers and adults. We've received hundreds of letters from customers who are thrilled with the results they've seen. Comments like "I'll never use anything else on my face" and "I finally feel pretty" are strong testimonials to the effectiveness of these natural alternatives for acne.

Natural relief for heartburn and acid indigestion

Common antacids have several side effects. Those containing aluminum can interfere with calcium and phosphorus absorption, and increase the body's exposure to an element that may damage brain cells. Those containing magnesium compounds can cause diarrhea when used in large doses, and should not be used by anyone with impaired kidney function. And the high sodium content in sodium bicarbonate antacids may lead to serious changes in the body's pH balance, which could negatively affect the heart and kidneys.

On the other hand, Enzymatic Therapy's **GastroSoothe®** contains calcium carbonate to help neutralize stomach acid without these dangerous side effects. Calcium carbonate is fast-acting and very safe, although it may cause constipation in large doses. GastroSoothe also contains deglycyrrhizinated licorice, a unique chewable extract widely used in Europe, and the amino acid glycine. GastroSoothe has no aluminum or sodium, and no added sugar or fructose. Its unique flavor may surprise you, but you'll definitely be pleased with the way it quickly relieves heartburn, indigestion, and sour stomach.

Natural relief for allergies, asthma, and sinus problems

Nasal sprays and antihistamines suppress nasal discharge, but the discharge is the body's way of getting rid of dead viruses, dead bacteria, dead white blood cells, and mucus. That's why Enzymatic Therapy designed Air-Power, As-Comp, AllerClear, and Sinu-Check for fast, natural relief of bronchial distress.

- **Air-Power**™ contains a powerful herbal expectorant, glycerol guaiacolate, which helps loosen phlegm and makes mucus thinner. Expectorants trigger productive coughs, helping to clear excess mucus out of the lungs and airways. While synthetic expectorants can cause nausea and drowsiness, glycerol guaiacolate does not. Air-Power also includes extracts of fenugreek seed, marshmallow, and mullein leaf.

- **As-Comp**™, an all-natural bronchodilator, temporarily relieves symptoms of bronchial asthma such as shortness of breath, tightness of chest, and wheezing. Its active ingredient, ephedrine, is a natural compound extracted from the Chinese herb ma huang *(Ephedra sinensis)*. Ephedrine works by relaxing the muscles surrounding narrow airways called bronchioles. This allows more air to flow into and out of the lungs.

  What sets As-Comp apart from synthetic asthma medications is its all-natural herbal base. Although we can only make health claims for its active ingredient, As-Comp also includes extracts of licorice root, marshmallow root (high in mucilage), goldenseal, ginger root, and other plants with a long history of use.

- **AllerClear**™ and **SinuCheck**™ are natural decongestants. They help clear nasal passages when they are blocked due to allergies (AllerClear) or colds and sinusitis (SinuCheck). The active ingredient in these formulas, pseudoephedrine HCL from *Ephedra sinensis*, is very similar to the one in As-Comp. Pseudoephedrine works by reducing swelling of the mucous membrane and suppressing the production of mucus. Like Air-Power and As-Comp, SinuCheck includes useful herbal extracts. AllerClear also contains a special formulation of essential vitamins and minerals, enzymes, glandular concentrates, and other natural factors.

Note: Whether synthetic or natural, ephedrine and pseudo-ephedrine can affect heart rate and should be used with caution, especially by anyone with heart problems, high blood pressure, or an overactive thyroid gland. Health-conscious individuals need to remember that even natural alternatives can have side effects and must be used as carefully and sensibly as their synthetic counterparts.

Natural relief for cold sores

Did you know that 80% of Americans over the age of 40 are infected with the virus that causes cold sores and fever blisters? Cold sores are one of the most widespread afflictions in the United States. They can be quite painful and frustrating, lasting up to two weeks. And they come back again and again whenever the right circumstances trigger the virus that causes them.

That's why Enzymatic Therapy searched the world to find a solution: **Herpilyn**™, a natural medicated cold sore cream. Herpilyn is manufactured by Lomapharm®, makers of Lomaherpan®, Germany's most popular natural cold sore product. Under an exclusive licensing agreement, Enzymatic Therapy is the sole distributor of Herpilyn in the United States.

Herpilyn's softening power can greatly reduce the severity of a cold sore, especially at the onset of its most annoying symptoms. European experience has conclusively shown that Herpilyn is incredibly effective when applied at the first tingling, itching, or burning experienced when a cold sore is coming on. Herpilyn is also very useful as an everyday lip balm for the relief of dry, chapped lips.

Herpilyn's active ingredient is allantoin, a natural compound derived from the comfrey plant. For topical use, comfrey has been a favorite of herbalists for over 2,500 years. Herpilyn also contains an extract of *Melissa officinalis* (lemon balm) concentrated at an unparalleled level of 70-to-1. No other cold sore product has this special 70:1 *Melissa* extract.

Herpilyn is completely nontoxic and safe for adults and children. Unlike some lip balms, it does not contain cortisone, which can have an adverse effect on cold sores. In addition, Herpilyn doesn't have the strong, unpleasant smell of other cold sore products.

Continually working on newer and better natural medicines

At Enzymatic Therapy, our work on new and better natural medicines keeps progressing. We continually search for innovative products that provide the most effective results. We are profoundly committed to developing and producing leading-edge products of the highest quality, based on substantial research and modern technology.

The demand for superior natural products and nutritional information keeps growing. More people are taking control of their health by improving their lifestyle and dietary habits, and by using nutritional and botanical supplements. More scientists and health care professionals are recognizing the link between nutrition and wellness. Enzymatic Therapy is proud to be a driving force in this new era of natural health.

Create your own nutritional plan

Now that you're familiar with the seven steps of enzymatic therapy, I'd like to show you how you can combine them to create your own nutritional plan for wellness. Each step has its advantage:

- Multivitamins provide general overall support, fortifying your diet with a well-rounded combination of all the essential vitamins and minerals your body needs.
- Antioxidants protect your cells against free-radical damage.

- Nutritional formulas provide the nourishment that specific body systems need to work properly in the long term.
- Glandular products support the function of your glands and organs.
- Herbal extracts contain natural compounds that target specific body tissues.
- Homeopathic remedies stimulate your body's self-healing mechanisms to take care of its symptoms.
- Natural OTC medicines provide quick, symptomatic relief of common health concerns.

Many people rely on more than one type of natural product to support their health. Some situations may call for the quick relief of a homeopathic remedy or natural OTC medicine. But to solve the underlying problem, proper nutrition is essential. And that's where a nutritional formula, glandular product, or herbal extract may help.

Here are several examples of how to combine the therapies for optimum results.

Enzymatic Therapy for Arthritis

Achy, stiff joints can turn everyday tasks—such as buttoning a shirt or turning a doorknob—into extremely painful chores for arthritis sufferers. The nutritional plan for arthritis combines therapies that relieve the pain and boost the intake of essential nutrients for the joints.

- *Homeopathic relief for the symptoms.* **Arthritis Remedy,** from Lehning Laboratories, is designed to relieve the aches, pains, and stiffness of arthritis, rheumatism, and sciatica (lower back pain). The all-natural homeopathic ingredients in Arthritis Remedy specifically help relieve arthritis pain in arms, elbows, fingers, joints, and knees.

- *Nutritional support for the joints.* Like all body tissues, joints need a constant supply of nutrients. Vitamin C, niacin, pantothenic acid, magnesium, manganese, zinc, and boron are especially important. Enzymatic Therapy's **ArMax**™ combines these essential nutrients with other natural compounds—including glucosamine sulfate—so your body can develop cartilage and other connective tissues important to the joints.

Cartilage is found where bones connect with other bones. Without cartilage, your bones would scrape against each other and you'd experience a lot of pain and inflammation. So you can see why it's important to get an adequate supply of the nutrients your body needs to make cartilage.

• *Glucosamine sulfate.* Vitamins and minerals aren't the only essential substances for healthy cartilage. A compound called glucosamine helps cartilage retain its gel-like nature and shock-absorbing qualities. When you supplement your diet with glucosamine sulfate, the most absorbable form of glucosamine, you support your body's natural process of cartilage production.

Glucosamine sulfate is available in the ArMax formula and by itself in **GS-500**. Whether you get your glucosamine sulfate in GS-500 or in ArMax, you can rest assured that we've done our homework. We chose to offer supplemental glucosamine sulfate for six reasons:

1. It is 98% absorbable, so more glucosamine gets to the joint structures.
2. It is supported by over 20 double-blind, placebo-controlled studies.
3. It is the preferred building block for connective tissue and cartilage.
4. Its sulfur components cross-link with other joint molecules for greater structural integrity.
5. Its simple molecular structure allows for quick, easy absorption. Glucosamine sulfate is far easier for the body to absorb than chondroitin sulfate, shark cartilage, and other cartilage extracts. The molecules in these formulas are 250 times larger

than glucosamine sulfate molecules. (That's a dramatic size difference! It's like trying to swallow a whole cantaloupe instead of a tiny sesame seed.)

6. It is the form of glucosamine recommended by researchers.

Enzymatic Therapy for Immune Function

The immune system works overtime when your body is battling a cold, the flu, or sinusitis. Most people take products that relieve the symptoms, but it's also vitally important to support immune functions.

- *Natural relief for the symptoms.* Homeopathic remedies such as **Cold & Flu Remedy** and **Sinus Remedy** from Lehning Laboratories can ease the coughing, sneezing, runny nose, aches, and itchy or watery eyes. Enzymatic Therapy's natural OTC medicines such as SinuCheck and Air-Power can help relieve the nasal and bronchial congestion associated with colds and sinusitis.

- *Nutritional support for the immune system.* Enzymatic Therapy's **ThymuPlex**™ provides essential vitamins and minerals for immune functions. This supplement combines antioxidants (vitamins A, C, and E, selenium, zinc) with thymus fractions, lysine, and herbal extracts.

  The thymus fractions are one of the key ingredients in this formula. They are low-weight molecular peptides and polypeptides broken down from whole thymus. These fractions are predigested to ensure a phenomenally high absorption rate of 95 to 98%. Enzymatic Therapy has the exclusive rights to these specially prepared thymus fractions, so you won't find them in any other company's supplement.

- *Herbal products.* Enzymatic Therapy's **Super Immuno-Comp** is designed for individuals who prefer an herbal supplement over a glandular one. This natural formula provides antioxidant nutrients with high-quality extracts of astragalus, echinacea, goldenseal, KS-2 (a polysaccharide from Shiitake mushroom), and licorice root. For people who rely on echinacea, our **EchinaFresh** provides the fresh-pressed juice of *Echinacea purpurea* in liquid and capsules (see pages 100 and 101).

Enzymatic Therapy for Prostate Function

Although the prostate gland is fairly small, it can cause big problems. That is why it's so important—especially for men over age 40—to get the proper intake of nutrients involved in sexual gland function.

- *Nutritional support for the male sexual glands.* Enzymatic Therapy's **PRO-50** combines vitamin A, zinc, and vitamin B6 with essential fatty acids, an amino acid complex, prostate tissue, and saw palmetto berry extract. Vitamin A, vitamin B6, and fatty acids are included because of their roles in hormone metabolism and sexual gland function. Zinc is especially important for prostate function. In fact, the prostate gland contains the highest concentration of zinc in a man's body.

- *Herbal products.* Many scientific studies have explored the link between saw palmetto berries and prostate function. For older men, researchers recommend 160 milligrams twice daily of a special liposterolic extract of saw palmetto berries. (A liposterolic extract is standardized for its content of fatty acids and sterols.) Each capsule of Enzymatic Therapy's **Super Saw Palmetto** provides 160 milligrams of this extract. For optimum natural benefits, it is standardized to contain 85 to 95% fatty acids and sterols—the level used in the studies.

Enzymatic Therapy for Stress

The nutritional plan for stress has two goals: relieve the symptoms of tension and anxiety, and boost the intake of essential nutrients that support body functions that deal with stress.

- *Homeopathic relief for the symptoms.* As mentioned in step 6 of this chapter, **Anti-Anxiety** from Lehning Laboratories safely relieves minor anxiety, nervous tension, and occasional stress.

- *Nutritional support for the body systems that deal with stress.* Enzymatic Therapy's **Stress-End** provides essential nutrients for the nervous system (the B vitamin complex), and for the adrenal glands (vitamin B6, pantothenic acid, vitamin C, and L-tyrosine). This formula also includes helpful minerals such as calcium, magnesium, potassium, manganese, and zinc with herbal extracts of valerian, passion flower, and Siberian ginseng.

What health concerns are you experiencing? Enzymatic Therapy can help. Explore your options; then create your own nutritional plan and take control of your health.

The information I've just shared with you may seem a bit overwhelming. Yet I believe that the more you understand natural products, the better chance you have of making intelligent choices. An informed person gets the most value for his or her money.

Choosing natural products isn't like picking out a shampoo or a garden hose or a car. You can replace your car, but you can't replace the human body. When you purchase natural products, you're making these choices for your most precious possession—your health. By choosing high-quality nutritional, glandular, and herbal supplements, homeopathic formulas, and natural medicines, you're investing in your most valuable resource.

If you have questions about the information in this chapter, or about any Enzymatic Therapy product, please call us toll-free at 1-800-783-2286.

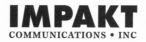

IMPAKT
COMMUNICATIONS • INC

P.O. Box 12496
Green Bay, WI 54307-2496
1-800-477-2995

ORDER FORM

Name: _____

Address: _____

City, State, Zip: _____

Phone Number: _____

BOOKS

❏ *Seven Keys to Vibrant Health* by Terry Lemerond ($10.95)

❏ *Breast Cancer* by Steve Austin, M.D. & Cathy Hitchcock, M.S.W. ($18.95)

❏ *Preventing & Reversing Osteoporosis* by Alan Gaby, M.D. ($16.95)

❏ *Questions & Answers on Family Health* by Jan de Vries ($10.95)

❏ *Healing Power of Herbs* by Michael T. Murray, N.D. ($17.95)

❏ *Natural Alternatives to Over-the-Counter and Prescription Drugs* by
   Michael T. Murray, N.D. ($30.00)

❏ *Encyclopedia of Natural Medicine* by Michael T. Murray, N.D. ($21.95)

❏ *Getting Well Naturally Series* (6 books) by Michael T. Murray, N.D.

   ○ *Arthritis*   ○ *Chronic Fatigue Syndrome*   ○ *Diabetes and Hypoglycemia*

   ○ *Male Sexual Vitality*   ○ *Menopause*   ○ *Stress, Anxiety & Insomnia*

   ($10.95 each) ○ All six for $60.00

❏ *Dr. Whitaker's Guide to Natural Healing* by Julian Whitaker, M.D. ($26.00)

MAGAZINE SUBSCRIPTIONS

❏ *Health Counselor* subscription ($18.00 for one year, $32.00 for two years)

❏ *Health Security* subscription ($12.00 for one year)

❏ *American Journal of Natural Medicine* subscription ($59.00 for one year)

METHOD OF PAYMENT

❏ Check   ❏ MasterCard   ❏ VISA   ❏ American Express

Name on card: _____

Signature: _____

Card number: _____ Exp. Date: _____